Journaling A Journey

Wendy Woolfson

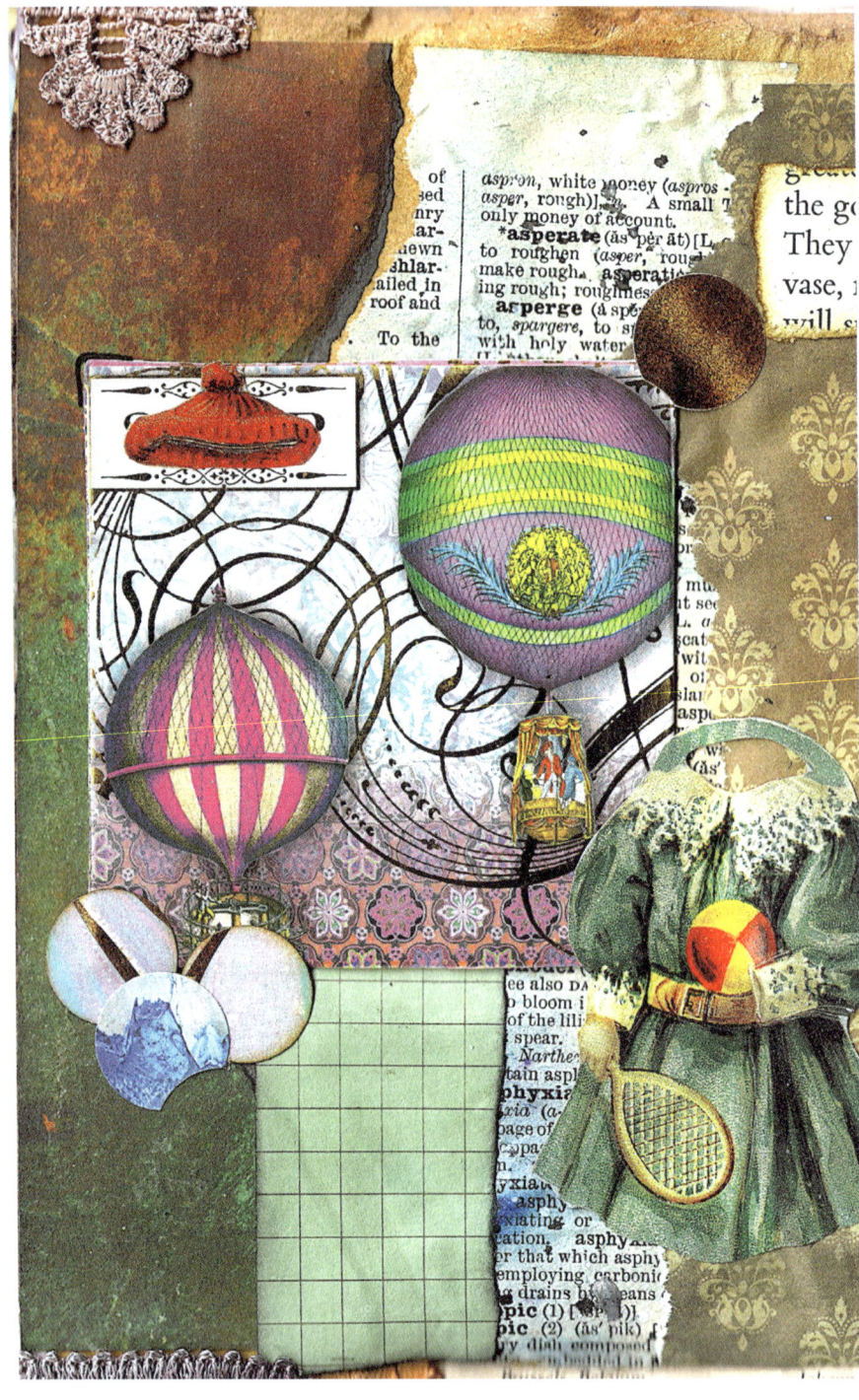

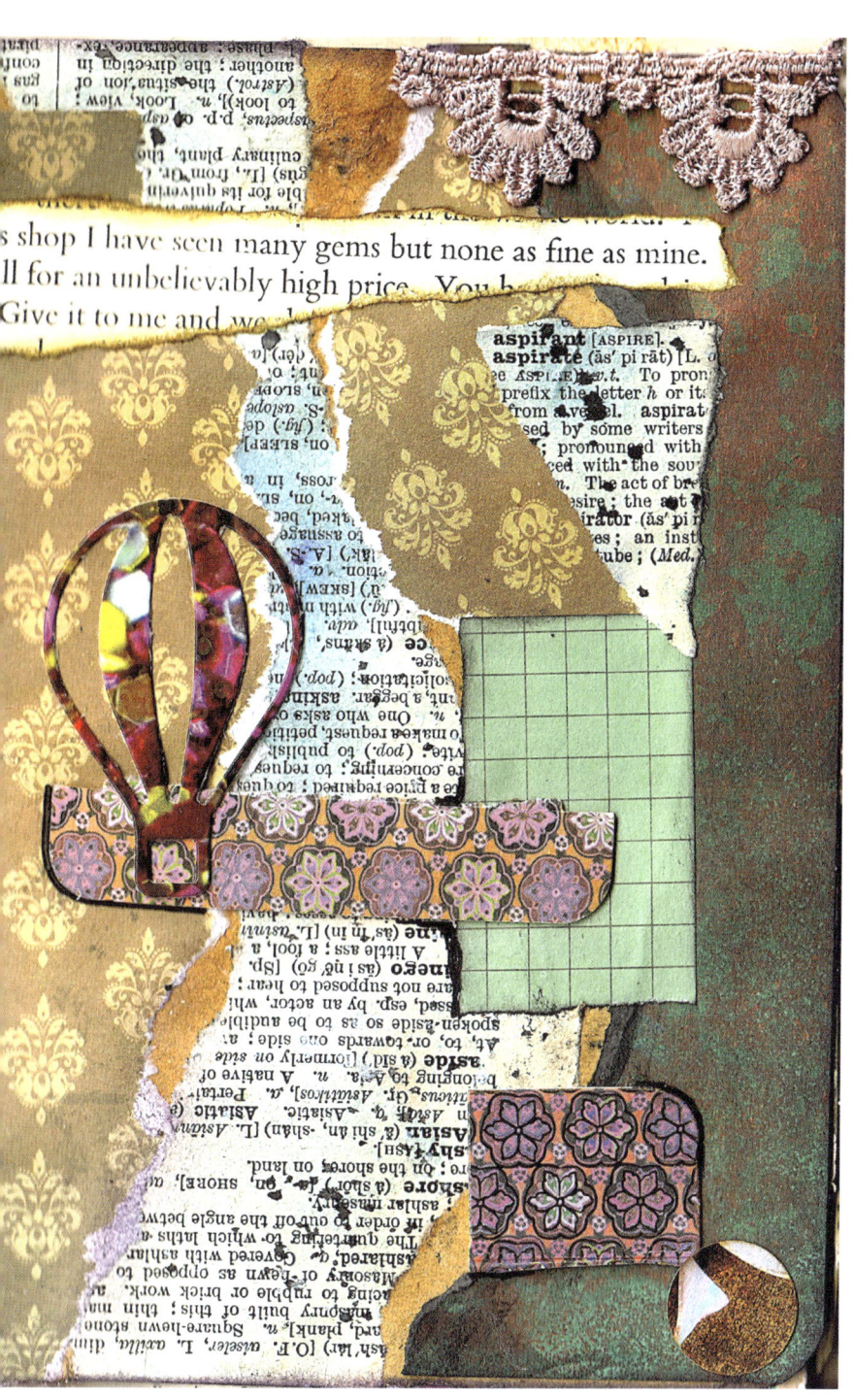

Words and artwork copyright © Wendy Woolfson March 2024

All rights reserved

No part of this bok may be reproduced, or stored in a retrieval system, or transmitted in any form or by any means, electronic, mechanical, photocopying, recording, or otherwise, without express written permission of the publisher

Dedication

To my husband Murray
whom I love with all of my heart

and my beautiful children
Harry and Angus
who will carry my heart
with them always

Contents

A Journey of a Thousand Miles Begins	1
The First Step	7
How To Be Sick	15
The Unbearable Certainty of the Uncertain	21
Healing From Trauma	27
A Helping Hand	33
All Is Not Lost	41
Fake It To Make It	47
Guardian Angel	55
Ink	63
Liminal Limbo	69
Open Up	75
The Diagnosis	85
The Piano	91
Pain	99
The System of Love	105
The Theory of Singing	113
Treatment and Recovery	121
The Motivation	129
About The Author ~ Wendy Woolfson ~	137
Acknowledgements	140
Thanks to ...	142
Journaling Pages	145
Support and Helplines	153
References	155
Transformation	160

14   MOLESWORTH'S POCKET-BOOK

To Cut the best Beam from a Log.

 Divide the diameter, $a\,b$, into 3 equal parts, $a\,f$, $f\,e$, and $e\,b$, and from e and f—draw the lines $f\,c$, $e\,d$, at right angles to $a\,b$— join $a\,c$, $a\,d$, $b\,c$, and $b\,d$, then $a\,c\,b\,d$ is the cross section of the beam required.

Strength of Rectangular Beams.
(Supported at both ends.)

B = Breadth of beam in inches.
D = Depth of ditto in inches.
S = Span of ditto in feet.
W = Breaking weight in cwt. at centre of beam.

$$W = \frac{B\,D^2}{S} \times K$$

K = 27 for wrought
 = 18 for cast i
 = 8 for cas
 = 6½ for

 = 7 fo
 = 6 fo
 = 5 f
 = 4
 = 3
 =
 = for

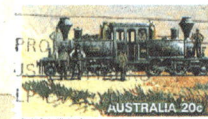

A Journey of a Thousand Miles Begins

"It is the greatest of all mistakes to do nothing because you can only do little, do what you can." Sydney Smith

This memoir covers the first six months following my diagnosis of stage 4 cancer. The book started as a blog on my newly updated website, and although I had planned on starting a blog at the time, I had no idea it was going to be chronicling my journey through cancer. In the end, the writing covered a range of topics from childhood trauma, mental health, spirituality and the intricasies of my diagnosis and treatment. The following are the updated and edited chapters which express what was happening for me at the time and how I processed it.

I have added an extra piece of writing to go with each chapter. I call this piece a Guided Message. It is what some people may also refer to as stream of consciousness writing, morning pages or channelled writing from our higher selves. Regardless of what any of us call it, I have found this way of writing to always be wiser than me and to have a very different voice from my own writer's style. The words are written without predicting what will come. They are entirely intuitive, and therefore for me an element I consider quite spiritual and connected with something bigger than myself.

The Guided Message provides an opportunity for you to reflect on your own circumstances and how the chapter that went before may impact on you and offer insight. It can also act as a stand-alone piece of writing that may contain some useful wisdom to apply to your own life.

My process for writing the Guided Message begins with taking a few deep cleansing breaths, and I drop into a more meditative state. I then put pen to paper or fingertips to keys, it doesn't matter which, and I allow whatever to come out just one word at a time. I don't predict what words will come. I keep my mind clear and just allow the flow of words. It's always so interesting as I have no idea what is going to come, and often I'm surprised at what is coming out! I'd like to invite you to have a go at this type of writing and I've provided a few pages at the back of the book for that purpose with some questions to prompt you. I have also included some notes pages at the end of some of the chapters to give you space for your own use.

Publishing this book has been cathartic to say the least. I spent the best part of my life living with trauma responses and not being at peace. It was only by going through a deep, therapeutic process that I gained the peace and self-awareness to write this book, something I had longed to do since childhood. I think the conversation around childhood trauma is still insufficiently acknowledged and I hope this book contributes something useful towards that. If I can find courage enough to write a second one, I will, although I know that book will be a much darker and more difficult task as it will tackle more personal and traumatic events.

Being a Professional Storyteller is another area that has supported me and brought me peace , and I am proud to be a part of the oral tradition here in Scotland. There are countless stories and storytellers that have supported me with their wisdom over the years, and I'm grateful to all of them.

There is one story that has always carried truth for me; the story of a farmer who seems to have bad luck continuously befall him. One night, his herd of horses are scared by a terrible storm and they run far off into the hills. His neighbours offer their commiserations at such bad luck, but the farmer just shrugs his shoulders and carries on saying, "We will see how it goes, nobody knows."

He sends his son out to fetch the horses back but in the process his son breaks his leg, and once again the neighbours come by and offer their disappointment at his bad luck, but the farmer shrugs his shoulders saying, "We will see how it goes, nobody knows."

His son is now no longer able to work in the fields or with the remaining few horses due to his injury, and they struggle for food and money. The neighbours offer their condolences at their misfortune and the farmer shrugs his shoulders and carries on saying, "We will see how it goes, nobody knows."

Soon after this, the Emperor declares that all the fit and healthy young men are to join the army to fight in an important war. The farmer watches as all the young men leave the village to go to war leaving his son behind. Again, the neighbours express their sadness and disappointment for the farmer that his son is unable to fight for the honour of their Kingdom, and the farmer shrugs his shoulders and carries on saying, "We will see how it goes, nobody knows."

Sadly, most of the young men do not return from the war or are seriously maimed in battle. Over time the son's leg mends, and they can return to prosperity with a fully functioning farm, and are then able to help and support the rest of the now struggling community.

His philosophy teaches us that none of us knows what the future may hold, and we need to have trust and hope that all will be well in one way or another.

I used to find that story so frustrating as in the early days I had what felt like very little in the way of hope. I didn't even understand the story or what hope meant. Now, I've learnt what it means, and I understand how to hold sway in the midst of terrible or troubling events, much like I find myself in now. I hope the stories in this book illustrate that, and they give hope to those who need it.

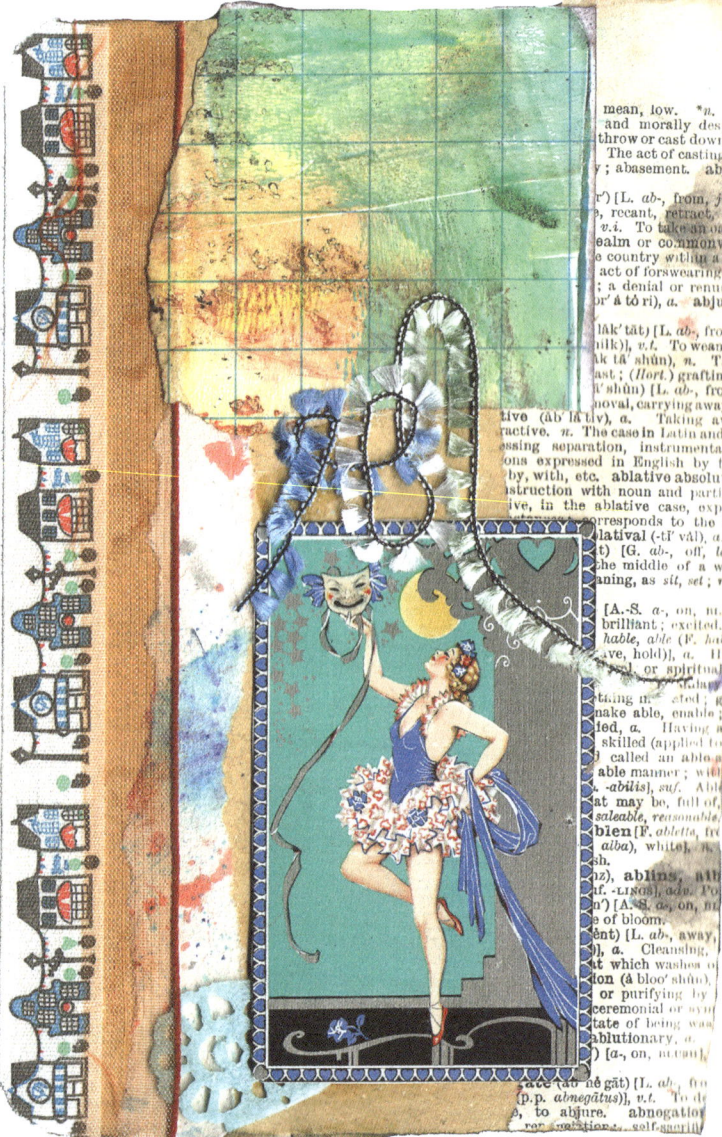

The First Step

Let's talk about the thing I never talk about, at least not on public forums like this; my personal experience of poor mental health and trauma. I've talked about it in different ways with friends, family, colleagues, in workshops, and people I've supported, but I've never got into it here before. It's such a huge subject to cover and I get exhausted merely thinking of writing about it but not as exhausted as I used to get, so that's why I'll talk about it now. I've decided now is the time to start writing about it, to draw a line under it, so to speak, and let the past go. Enough time has passed, and enough healing been done to support me to open up. I have good boundaries, something I put a lot of value on and have worked hard to learn about and put in place. I also want to share because I hope my story might help someone else. This is just a small piece, and I may or may not write more as this will be a processing experience for me as well.

It took until I was forty-six years old to pluck up the courage to ask for help. By the time I did I was feeling suicidal every day. I was self-harming in a variety of ways, and I could feel no emotions, I only felt numb. I was

THE FIRST STEP

walking through my days like a zombie, crying when no-one was looking, drinking too much, and doing zero to look after myself. I had started to make plans for killing myself and I had no idea how to break the cycle and ask for help; except that I did know how to do that, but asking for help felt like it wasn't an option. It made me feel too vulnerable, something I was not prepared to feel. If I asked for help then someone would ask me what I needed help with, and what was wrong, and that question was so huge I had no idea how to answer it. If just one small brick were to be taken out of the wall I had so meticulously built over the years, well, I just couldn't bear the thought of what might happen. But each day had become so painful. I felt I was dragging my feet through clay, and the cracks were beginning to show.

   I was driving home one night, and I was approaching the counselling centre which I passed regularly on various commutes, I knew I had to pull in. I had been building up to this for several weeks. The thought had been drifting around in my head, nagging away at me like a mini counsellor sitting on their chair with a notebook saying, 'Wendy, you know if you were talking to someone who told you they were feeling this way you would suggest it would be helpful for them to talk to someone and seek out some therapy.'

I parked the car and walked through the front door towards the lift, being careful not to catch anyone's eye and get drawn into any awkward conversations or questions. I got out at the second floor, walked up to the unstaffed desk, and waited. Eventually, someone arrived, and I heard myself asking if I could please refer myself for some counselling. They put me on their waiting list, and I walked out of there with a small sense of achievement and, if I admitted it, a small weight lifted too. I knew the waiting list was long, but I also knew I had done an important thing and tethered myself to a piece of hope. I still stopped at Tesco though and bought a bottle of red wine for when I got home.

Walking into that counselling centre was a key moment because it probably saved my life. Even just knowing that I was on a waiting list was enough to give me reason to live; the thought that I might soon have an outlet to share some of the terrible thoughts in my head. Don't let a waiting list put you off, ever.

The tricky thing then was managing life while I was waiting for a counsellor, and it took all my strength to carry on. Never underestimate how hard someone with mental health problems is working just to function in everyday life. At that time, I had worked in and around mental health for about seven years, and I'd studied a broad range of models and methods of support and

THE FIRST STEP

worked in various settings. That's how I knew that I was going to be the only person to save me. I was drowning and nobody else knew it because I was brilliant at hiding it. Every day I put on my mask and presented myself to the world and every night I fell apart. How did I do that? I guess in the first place it was my passion for my work. I knew the people I supported needed me and they were my priority. It also worked as a distraction from my own troubles. Over the years I've learnt that spending a couple of hours with a young person always leaves me feeling a hundred percent better than I was feeling before. Young people can have that effect on you, and if there's one thing I love to do, it's help people with their problems, especially young people. I can still relate to them and step into my own teenager's shoes and remember what it was like, that really helps.

    I had my other moments too; I'm one of those people who, when they cry, their face recovers quickly and doesn't stay blotchy and red for more than a minute. So, I could silently cry in the toilet or in my car and emerge fresh faced with no-one knowing the difference. I buried myself in my work and started journaling every day. I carried a notebook and pen with me everywhere I went and wrote whatever I needed. I had a separate book by my bedside and at night I filled it with all the darkest thoughts I knew I couldn't share with anyone: it was my silent counsellor.

JOURNALING A JOURNEY

It can be strange when you're the person supporting others with their mental health problems and all the while you're falling apart yourself. Fortunately, my story has a happy ending which is not something I would have predicted back then, and I hope by sharing pieces of it here it will provide hope for those who are struggling and insight for those who need it.

Please don't struggle with your mental health on your own. Reach out to a friend or family member if you can, or sometimes talking to a stranger is easier. At the end of the book are a few numbers you can call for good, confidential support.

Notes

Guided Message

It takes a huge amount of strength to be the one to help and save yourself, and it is not to be underestimated. You were sinking into the depths of despair that would destroy you and you had the wherewithal to recognise this. What more can anyone do in desperate times except what they can? Never berate yourself for all the negative things you do to yourself or that you have done because all of it has a purpose in one way or the other and will get you to where you need to be in the end. So, as we always say, everything happens perfectly and in perfect time. There is no need to panic or to doubt oneself, only to rest in our arms of reassurance and trust that if you listen, we will guide you to the next best step. That next step might not always look obvious or even appear to be the best choice but if you put your faith in it then it will surely get you to where you need to be. Be strong in your decisions and remember we have always got your back.

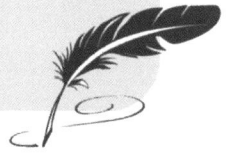

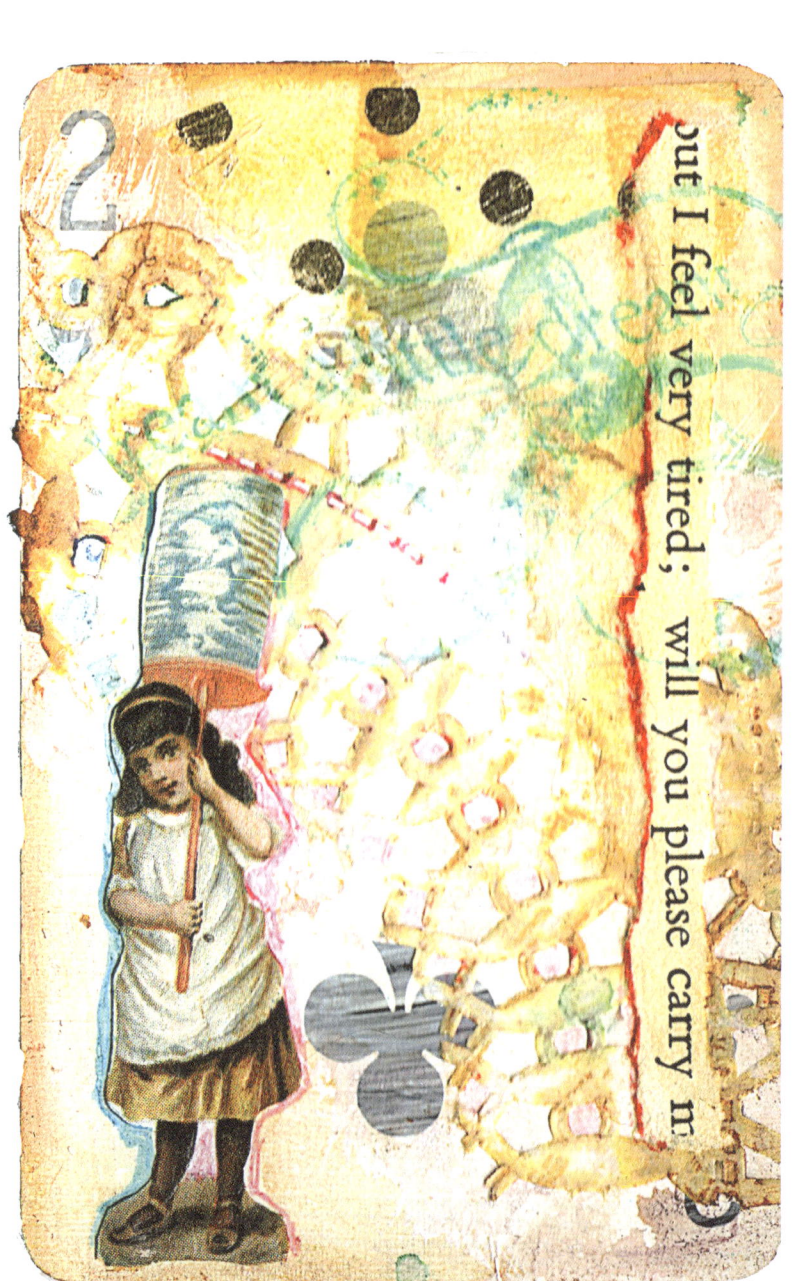

How To Be Sick

Before I was ill the most medication, I'd ever taken was a couple of paracetamol and ibuprofen and the occasional course of anti-biotics. Then I have cancer, and overnight my dressing table turns into a pharmacy.

I have pills spilling over the edges; anti-inflammatories, nerve pain killers, opiates, constipation pills, steroids, paracetamol, a daily nasal rinse, and anti-sickness pills to help with the effect all the other pills have on me. Oh, the irony.

I've made mistakes with the quantities I'm taking as well, either taking too many or too few.

Nobody tells you how to do this properly.

How to be sick.

How to manage all this medication and understand it. It all happens so quickly, and the professionals throw all this information at you almost as soon as you receive the diagnosis, and just like that, my whole life has changed from running a service in social care with a team of nine and a caseload of hundreds to just, nothing. I am now the priority and medicine my main focus.

Measurements, milligrams, and quantities.

When to take these ones, how many of those, and at what time of day.

Opiates twice a day, nerve pills 3 x a day, anti-sickness 3 x a day (because the nausea is constant)

Bowel relaxant powder sachets as and when required – how much am I supposed to poo in a day, is there a required amount?

A phone call with the pain management nurse regarding the breakthrough opiates. Me, "Oh, one syringe of 5ml equals 10mg? I thought two syringes equals 10mg?" which means they think I've been in much less pain than I have, and I've been in in a lot more pain than they understood. Nurse, "Let's increase your tablet opiates then." Thank God, I finally get a night's sleep with no pain after three months.

They throw you into this world of medicines and measurements and assume that you're going to understand and cope with it all, whilst in pain and exhausted. I'm no Ginger Rodgers, I can't do this whilst wearing heels and backwards, (you might be too young for that one). I struggle with numbers and measurements as it is, so this just pushes the limits of what I can deal with whilst swallowing 160mg of Morphine per day.

I have a pill box for Monday to Sunday, 4 x a day all laid out so I can't get it wrong. But I still do. I still run out and forget to re-order the repeats from the surgery and then it's a scramble to get the chemist and surgery to line up their systems and help me get my pain meds on time.

We bought them a box of chocolates to thank them for their help.

My husband helps with all this of course but whilst holding down his job, looking after the boys, keeping the household together, looking after me and running to the surgery and chemist for various prescriptions. When I look at all the things he must do, then what I'm going through, it starts to pale in comparison, and I'm exhausted for him.

The doctor phones as I'm writing this with the news of the upcoming Oncology appointment, a word that now appears easily on my phone's predictive text, to remind me to take the time to ask all the questions I need, and he tells me he's never seen a diagnosis like this in all his career. I get emotional. This is the man who was the one to recognise there was something wrong with me months ago. If it wasn't for him, I think I'd still be waiting for that elusive ENT appointment. I thank him again for his help through deep breaths and sobs. It's time for a shower and to wash away fear. There's still living to be done.

Guided Message

How remarkable humans are that they can juggle all of this! You continue to put one step in front of the other each day and remain focused on your great task of healing. Do not give up for you are more than capable, you only need to look at how far you have come and the life that stretches behind you to see all you have achieved, and why not be proud of that? So, this in the big map of your life may be only a small blip, and within time you will have mastered the meds and overcome your illness. Regardless of outcomes, though, you must see yourself as invincible and highly skilled in your own life. You know best what you need and can look out for yourself. Do not view yourself as weak, courageous one, because you are facing great challenges, and it is your lion strength that will get you through. All paths lead to healing in one way or another and we welcome and celebrate you in all ways whatever the outcome. Stand firm as you reach out for all the things you need and remember to always ask for help when it is needed. People love to give and when you allow them to help it is a gift to them to do so. You are not doing this alone, you were never meant to do this alone, so welcome in your friends and family to join you on this great adventure.

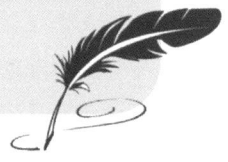

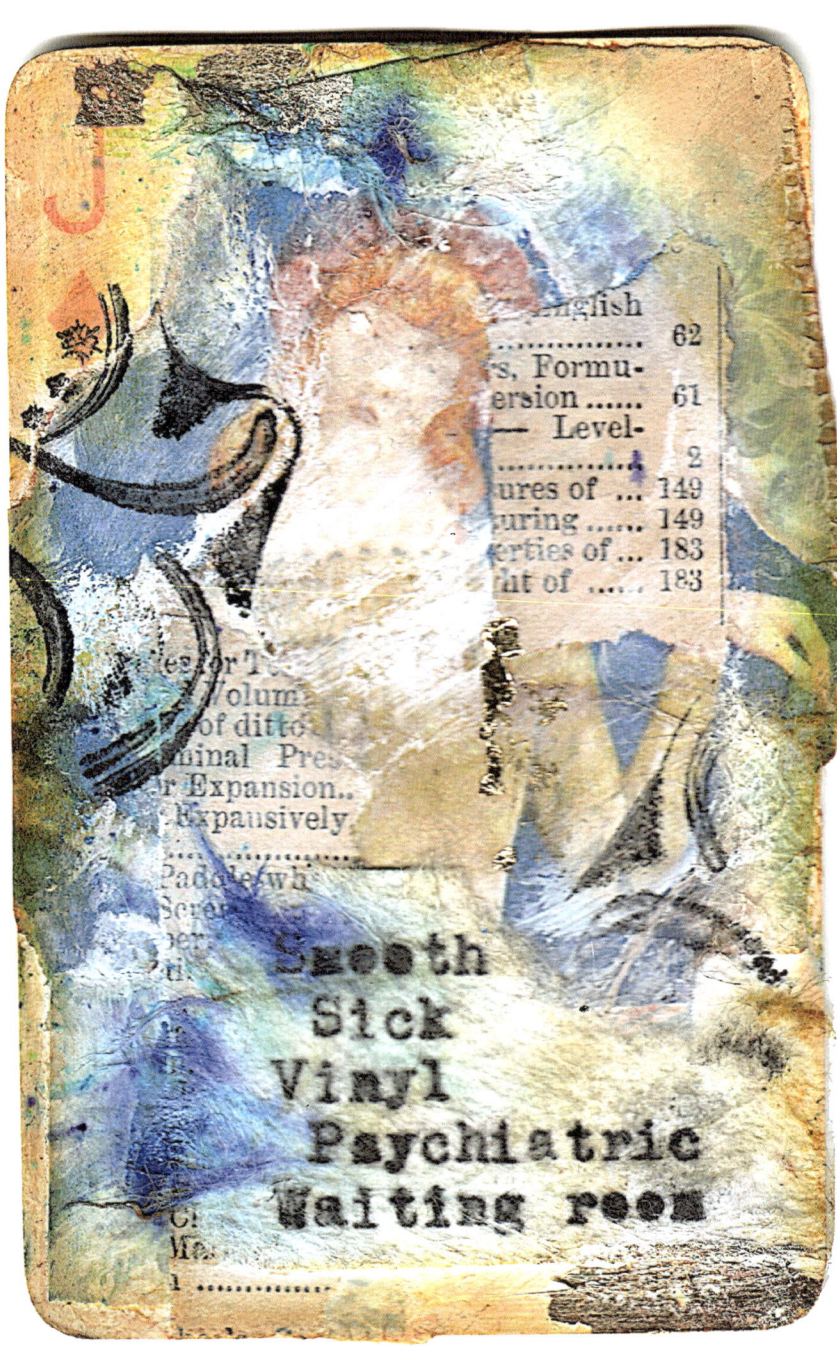

The Unbearable Certainty of the Uncertain

I've never been in this place before where the uncertainty is so certain. Where I know I will not know anything for weeks and yet I can be certain I'll be in some level of pain for that whole time.

I am in a holding place of pain where my head feels like it's in a vice half the time and the other half like my face is on fire, and then the intolerable moments when it's all happening at once. The nerves are on edge, quite literally, and there is nowhere else for me to go except the medicine cabinet for the kind of hardcore drugs that usually one would have to score off someone on the street. Thankfully, the drugs work.

My mood is dipping low this week as I have a post-op nosebleed and oedema in the lower half of my body, both of which only decide to show up at the weekend when I can't phone anyone to find out what's going on. Doctor Google must suffice, and I need to do my

THE UNBEARABLE CERTAINTY

best to stay away from the obvious scary articles and stick to the descriptions of pain med side effects and trust to common sense that it's all quite normal, even though it feels awful. My mood dips ever lower as the end is not even in sight. The end is in fact a complete unknown factor that may come later rather than sooner as so far, the NHS has not been rushing to push through preliminary investigations, with my urgent ENT appointment having taken six months to fulfil.

In the meantime, I've stuck my head in the sand and completely ignored the reality of what has so obviously been growing inside my head for the last eighteen months. A tumour, which I believe is filled with all my childhood and adult trauma, of which there has been much. I saw the image of it on the MRI scan. It hung there like a strange fruit, the harbinger of doom hanging from the nerve that separates the cavity of my skull from my brain, a white line neatly surrounding it, like someone just drew it there for fun, as though a child had outlined it in a wobbly line of white crayon. It looked so neat and tidy in its white balloon bubble, but I know, I know in my heart it holds all my secrets, and all my pain. I thought I'd got away with it, no serious diagnosis for me, just three and a half years of trauma therapy and then boom, I drop the mic and walk away. I'm all done, and life is sweet.

Life really has been sweet the last few years. I finally reached a point in my life where I'm happy and we have a rhythm and routine and for the most part, it's all good, and then this happens. It's messed up man. Yet, at the same time, I know exactly why this has happened, because everything wasn't all good. I had been ignoring my dreams, again. I did that once before twenty years ago, and the same thing happened, the universe launched an offensive and turned my whole world upside down to get my attention, so I'd have to look at it.

So that's what I'm doing, I'm looking at it, I'm re-evaluating my life.

For now, I will take each day as it comes and embrace the uncertainty that this challenge brings. I've been in dark places before, and I've learnt how to cope. In recent years I've met good people and I've learnt how to ask for help, and that will get me through. That, and everything my life has taught me up until this very moment.

I am certain I will recover.

Notes

Guided Message

You have identified what you need to do and what you need. And that is a massive step forward from the way things used to be. You recognise how you are feeling and actions you can take, as well as accepting where you are. Dear child, when we are faced with difficulties of such enormity it is normal for us to go 'offline' so to speak, and lose our direction, that's ok. What is important is to not lose ourselves, and this is something you are determined not to do, and we commend that. A positive outlook can help so much in recovery, and this is no different. Step forward into your diagnosis and feel what is to be done, each step of the way. There is no right or wrong, only the action of the moment, and that, my friend, is the wonder of this uncertainty.

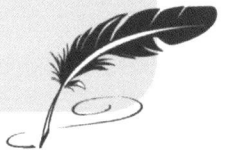

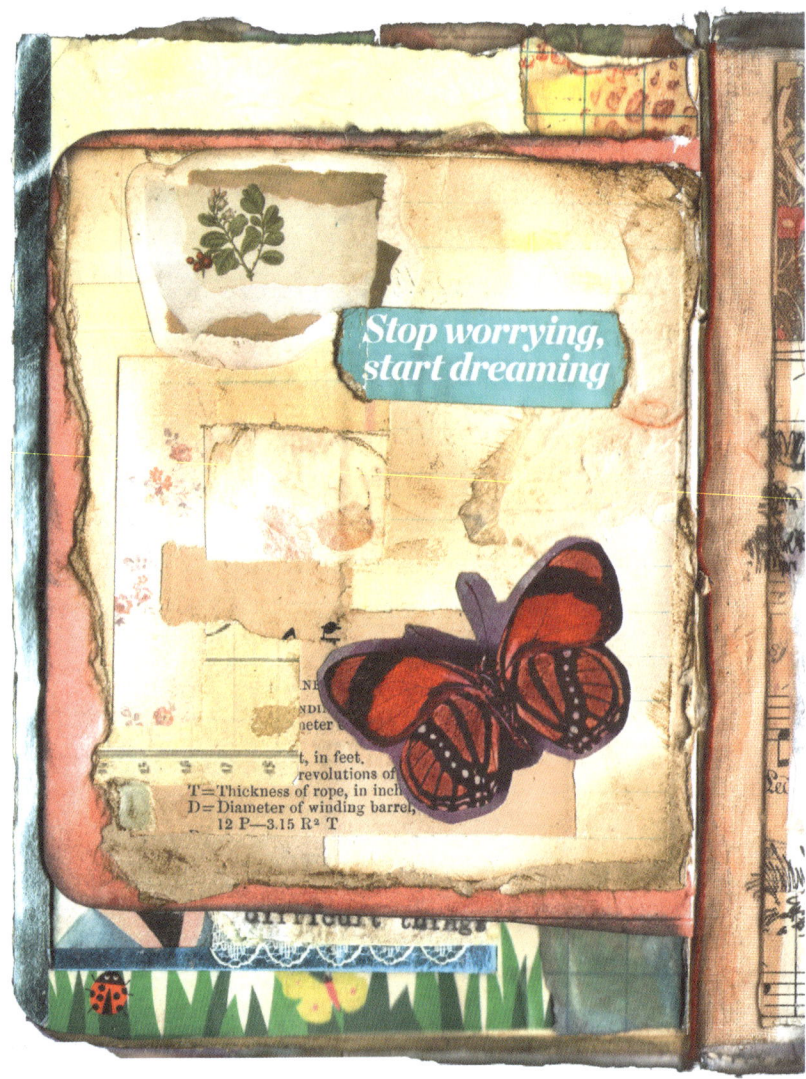

Healing From Trauma

I've had a lot of traumas in my past and it's done now. It's done. But now I'm sick.

Now, I'm healing, and that's different work. There's been self-reflection and inner work, studying Reiki, and deep spiritual practice. I had three and a half years of successful trauma therapy for a diagnosis of Complex Post Traumatic Stress Disorder (CPTSD). And I made it through even when I thought I never would. Even when I really thought, this is it, I'm done here. But I was lucky, I had kids, and they kept me going. I had a husband to love and support me.

When I was about fifteen, I was sitting with my friends in Shawlands Arcade eating our packed lunches during school lunch break, and feeding the pigeons, and we were talking about our future. We were imagining the year 2000, when we'd be thirty and what we would be doing, wondering what would life and the world be like. At the time I couldn't think what thirty would be like, but I had a strong sense of what fifty was. I remember saying, everything will come right for me when I'm fifty, that's when I'm going to study something different or be successful or whatever. It felt like I was making a prophecy and the feeling inside me was strong. I just knew in my heart that that was the age when my life would get good or come right. That doesn't say much for the intervening years, but we'll get to that another time.

Well, here I am at fifty-two, and I'd say that fifteen-year-old Wendy was right. I never forgot what I said. It was one of those things that would come up now and again in my life, and I'd remember I'd said that, and I'd have a fleeting memory of what it felt like sitting on that cold bench on a cold, grey day and, in a weird way, it would keep me going.

I was in my forties when I hit my rock bottom, and I remembered it then, thank God, and it gave me a kind of hope because I'd made it that far even when I thought I wouldn't. I wasn't wrong either. It's not that everything before that was bad, just that it was always an internal struggle. I hadn't dealt with my demons from the past, and there were legions of them. My heart and my body felt broken, and all used up. I didn't know how to live comfortably in my own body and in this life, it was a constant struggle.

Now, here I am, facing another struggle but of a different kind and I don't see it as traumatic, not like the things I've faced in the past. I see this as healing. I see this illness as the residual result of all I have been through, the physical expression of it all. I will help it heal because it's been through a lot, and it needs my care. Like a bully, fighting it will only make it stronger, so I will love it instead. I will hold it in my arms and cry for all it's been through and witnessed, and I will come out the other side a renewed and different person.

Notes

Guided Message

Dear child you have so much courage and every word you say to yourself is true. You have bigger dimensions inside of you than you can even imagine, and your capacity to heal is strong and is huge. When you can view your illness as an ally rather than enemy then you begin the healing process. You need to stay steady and focused like an anchor, and not scattered like the wind. Surround yourself in love and give yourself all the love you need, and that is a lot. You are healing generations in this lifetime; you all are as you are the new generations come to bring healing to this planet through your own healing. Every time you heal an issue in your life it adds to the light of this world, and you all shine a little brighter. Do not despair because brighter days are returning and as long as you remain focused, all will be well.

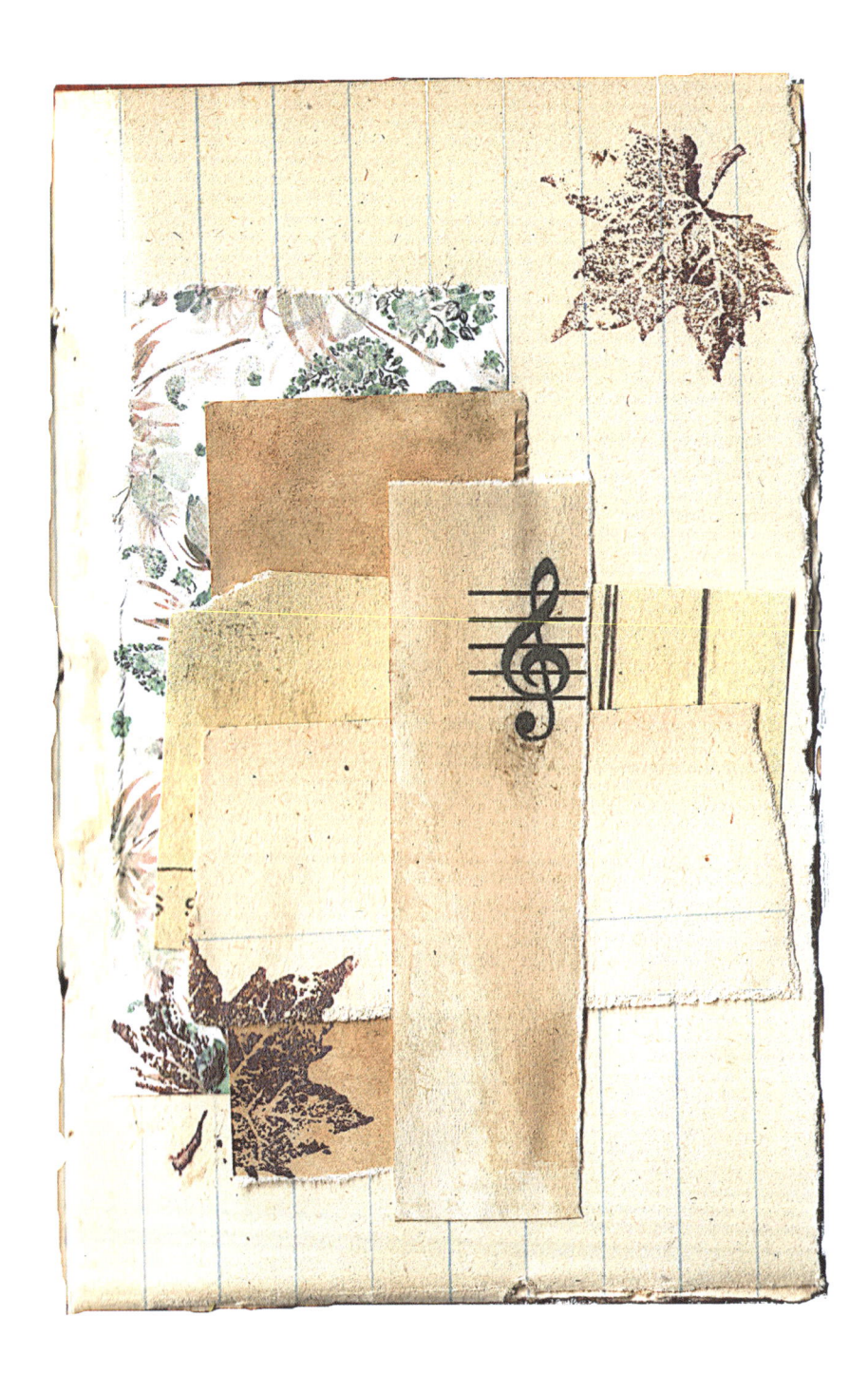

A Helping Hand

Asking for help is vital for survival.

If we look at Maslow's hierarchy of needs, we see all the things that he considered are vital for humans to survive and grow, and at the very foundation of that is food, shelter, and warmth. He suggested that if they are not present the child won't survive. It's also been generally recognised more recently that fundamentally it's not enough; we also need love and compassion.

"If just food, shelter, clothing and education filled all of a child's needs, orphanages would be ideal parents", Peg Streep, from her book Daughter Detox

There's not always an adult around to spot that a child is in difficulty, so being able to ask for help is an important skill and needs to be taught as it's one that many do not have. For some reason our society has draped a cloak of shame over asking for or needing help. I think these days our children are expected to grow up much more quickly than they ever have, and to feel like they ought to be more responsible and resilient than they are. However, if a child is taught to ask for help then even in the direst situation they can be saved. This comes back again to having a loving adult in their life, and by that, I mean someone who is looking out for them with a sense of love, compassion, or care. This doesn't only have to be a parent but a teacher or a family friend too. Someone who notices them and reminds them they can ask for help and that if they do, they will be believed, listened to, and supported. It's an incredibly powerful protective factor, especially in cases of abuse.

I felt I couldn't ask for help from the earliest age. I always thought I should just somehow know the answer to everything, to all my problems and because I didn't, then I must be a failure. This was not because I was egotistical, although it is connected to ego but in a different way, it was more a lack of self-esteem, I just couldn't admit it. I thought it was weak and meant I showed a lack of strength and courage. If I couldn't do something myself or know how or what needed to be done, then I was 'less than' and not good enough. That's a hard way to live your life and why it's vital to instil in children the idea of working as part of a team and that helping each other is good. We can also model this for them by asking for help in our own daily lives to remove any stigma.

If I hadn't learnt this well enough before, then the cancer has certainly taught me that now, and I've asked for and accepted levels of assistance I never even knew existed for me.

Friends and family have gone beyond what I could have even imagined in the ways they have helped me, and my family and I know it benefits all of us. We've all learnt so much from me having cancer. In no particular order I've learnt humility, gratitude, patience, what's important and what isn't, how much I love people, and how much other people love me, being still, strength, and handling pain.

I've seen my husband put all my needs first without a grudge or being annoyed, but with an unthinking desire to care for someone he loves. We talked about how he's learnt what caring for someone involves and that he's stronger and more resilient than he thought. We can see how important friends and family are and how wonderful it is that they have stepped up without hesitation, and with generosity to do whatever they can.

We know now what cancer really means: an incredibly tough journey emotionally, mentally, and physically, and how it really affects people.

A HELPING HAND

My husband has been reflecting on how important the community is, including the local surgery, and especially the staff at the local chemist who go out of their way to do whatever they can. It's lovely how they know everybody in our wee town, and we can see that they're an important hub here. It's nice to have friendly people looking out for you. In a small town like we live in, people remember you and know your face and they try to help you because they know you're suffering and want to help.

Most of all, we've come to know exactly how much we love each other, and that our love is stronger than ever. What a wonderful thing to have to come out of this. We're very lucky.

I love asking for help now, and I can see that when we ask for any kind of guidance, we are offering someone the gift of an opportunity to ease a situation for another, and to provide support if they can. It's a gift, because helping someone who is in need gives us a sense of pleasure and satisfaction, and why would we limit that for anyone? Help can come in all different guises and there's no need to enforce a restriction on what we think aid might look like.

I used to become very fixated on how I thought things should be. I had this need to control situations to make me feel safe. I had ideas about what certain things should look like or how they should play out, and it was all wrong. It was all so distorted by my poor mental health and skewed world view. During therapy my layers of bravado and ego were gently removed, and I was encouraged to see clearly how important it is to reach out to people and ask them for their help. I could see how pleased that made them feel that someone would think of them as capable of being of assistance in my difficult situation, and the joy that could potentially bring, even when someone is suffering, and that's ok, it's as it should be, we should be happy we can help when someone is in need.

That is what the quote at the start of this book is about. I used to be so scared of offering any help to others at all because I felt what I could offer was so puny and worth so little. Now I realise that it's the smallest of gestures that can mean more than anything and be the thing to make the biggest difference.

So, I have shed those layers of fear and allowed the truth to be revealed, and what a difference it has made to my life. I'm eternally grateful to everyone who has helped me on my journey, and I hope I can repay it to them someday or as is now common to say, I can 'pay it forward' meaning, I do something to help another

A HELPING HAND

person instead, or as well. I mean, why not just help everyone without thinking about it anyway?

There is so much pain in the world right now, so much war and discord in almost every area, that we need each other and our communities more than ever. I hope we can all become much more caring and loving towards each other in all ways and do it without giving it a second's thought, and together we will all create a more compassionate world, helping one person at a time.

Guided Message

Humble yourselves not before a god or a higher power but before your own self, for you are indeed your highest power. It is you who you give the greatest thanks to, and when you give help to another being you are giving of your whole self which is an incredibly deep and loving act. This concept of proffering assistance to another is overcomplicated and one need only step forward with a kind word or hand at any time to conduct an act of God. Rejoice in your success as you change another's life merely by a small act of kindness. This is what changes the whole world and as you have said is what is needed right now. Go forth and enjoy all that is on offer and be the one that makes that change. It is all in the palm of your hand and on the tip of your tongue. In your own ways you are gods for you may hold the fate of another's happiness or even safety in your command. Do not hesitate to help when you see it and always make amends when you can.

Light cracks
against the dark

1935.

All Is Not Lost

I remember the first time I found the skeleton of a leaf. It was under a huge, low tree with long, spreading branches. I can't remember what kind of tree it was, but I was about eight years old, and I was hiding under there during a game of hide and seek. It was surprisingly dark with shapes of sunlight dropping through the close branches, creating interesting patches of light on the ground.

I looked down, and there at my feet I saw something that I never knew existed. It looked impossible, and in the half light, I thought it was. I bent down to pick it up and then I could see it was the skeleton of a leaf. As it dawned on me what it was it just blew my mind. Firstly, I had no idea that leaves even had a skeleton that would survive after they rotted away, and secondly, I wondered what the skeleton was for, why was it even there? I marvelled at how long the leaf must have lain on the ground in all kinds of weather, for there to be nothing left but this thin, fragile frame.

I sat down in the musty scented humus, the soft, deep, carpet floor of years of fallen leaves, woven through the dust and detritus of small forest animals. If I dug deep enough into it, who knows what I might find.

Carefully, I picked up and gently held this immensely fragile skeleton of a leaf in the small palm of my hand and tried to understand how long it had been there. To me, it was the most beautiful thing I had ever seen and holding it in my hand felt like a privilege. I lifted my head and looked around me at the ground I was sitting on. I saw more skeleton leaves just like the one I held in my hand, and I wanted them all. I wanted to collect as many as I could and take them all home so I could look at them whenever I wanted to. I started to pick them up but as I placed them together in a small bundle in my little hand, which was beginning to sweat a little, they began to disintegrate. They started to become tangled with each other and clump and fall apart, I tried hard to salvage them, but I only made it worse with the clumsiness of my child fingers. The ones I had put in my pocket had turned to dust. I was heartbroken. I looked around to find another one that was as good as the first one I found, but I was distracted by the call of my friends and someone finding me.

I have never forgotten that day, and since then, whenever I go for a walk in the woods I have a look for a skeleton leaf, and if I find one, I am eight years old again and sitting under that spreading tree on my own in the half light, marvelling at the impossible magic and fragility of what I hold in my hand.

With the detritus of those decades behind me, I am comforted by the belief that anything is possible and, over time, all that we are will return to the warmth of the earth, but the beautiful, impossible bones of us will always remain to remind those left behind of the beauty that once existed.

Notes

Guided Message

Dear one, how special to sit underneath the branches of an ancient tree and feel its wisdom. There is much to be learnt from nature and much to be felt. Great healing comes from being surrounded by nature and all that she offers. The earth is abundant with life in all the smallest of places, the hidden and the depths as described. The layers of the earth exude such strength to enable you to be supplemented by her when needed. You need only go out to sit or walk in nature to feel replenished. Even gazing at nature from your window can offer healing and there is no wrong way to interact with her. Enjoy the gifts that surround you and savour what has been gifted to use freely to aid your life. There is great wisdom in the plants and herbs, be stimulated by them and enjoy!

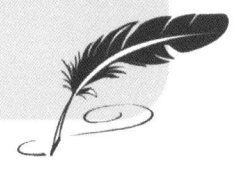

MINDFUL
THINKING

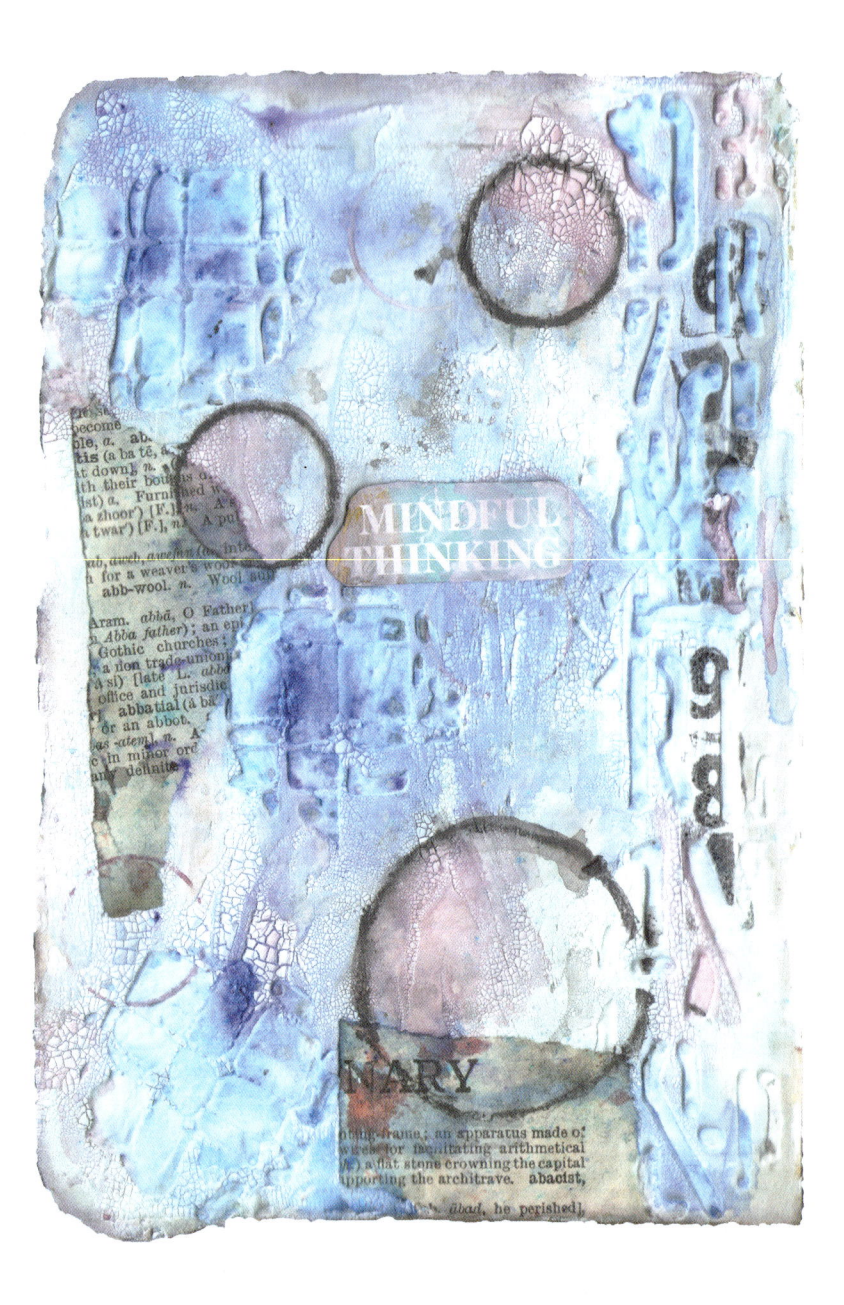

Fake It To Make It

I'm sitting in a café at the Beatson as I write this. The Beatson is the main cancer treatment centre in Glasgow, and a place I'm getting more familiar with on each visit. It's not somewhere I enjoy attending, and it does not make me happy.

Lately, the topic of joy has been coming up, so I thought I would have a look at it. It's not something I've ever properly understood or explored but I'll do my best.

I know someone who runs laughter workshops and whose business it is to bring joy to others and help them to become more joyful in their lives. I admire them greatly. I attended one of their workshops many years ago, and I remember I found it extremely difficult and exhausting. During the session one of the things we did was fake laughing; the idea that by pretending to laugh it would lead to a sensation of happiness and real laughter. As we got into it, I could see that the other participants were getting a lot out of it, but I found it really hard to do. I did genuinely laugh at times, but I also felt exhausted and strained. I like to laugh as much as anyone else but if you asked me if I experienced joy in that moment, I would have to say no. That's no reflection on the workshop or the facilitator, that's just me, I didn't understand what joy was or what it was meant to feel like.

I thought of joy as being loud and exuberant, an extrovert emotion that causes a huge feeling of elation. I was also going through a tough time in my life, and it was simply bad timing. I didn't understand the purpose of the work and I still had much to learn about joy.

I went to that workshop because I was unhappy and I wanted to change how I felt by experiencing joy, this elusive thing that I could never quite grasp. I also believed, and still do, that the world needs more joy in it, and that if we start with us, it spreads. I wonder if you've seen the video of a man standing in a busy train carriage, and he starts to laugh, quietly at first, and then a bit louder, seemingly laughing at something funny to himself. But the more he continues to laugh, the people beside him begin to laugh too and very quickly the whole carriage is laughing and smiling with each other. It's beautiful to watch and I couldn't help but laugh as I was watching, and I'm even smiling as I type this and remember it. It's true, laughter is contagious.

They say that laughter is the best medicine, and who knows if that is true, but I know I always feel better after I've had a good laugh about something. It lifts my energy and my spirits. I'm still smiling as I write this because I'm writing about laughter and smiling, isn't that funny?

When I was going through therapy, I barely lifted the corners of my mouth. I had lost the will to even try to be happy. I can remember looking at people who were laughing and smiling and hating them, whilst not understanding how they could be so happy. I kept asking myself, where did that laughter come from? What was making them so happy? I was lost and all I could see was the darkness and no light. I couldn't be bothered trying to be happy, it needed too much energy, like in the laughter workshop, it was exhausting to laugh. For me, there was no point left in life. As far as I could see there was nothing to feel happy about. I really did just want to die.

Gradually, as therapy continued and the years passed by, I began to feel better, and as that happened, I started to notice the lighter things in life. I can't remember exactly how or when it happened, but I can remember it started with music.

FAKE IT TO MAKE IT

I decided I was going to listen to different music, something uplifting. I had been listening to a lot of dark and sad music, which had fitted my mood but now that I recognised I was starting to feel better it was time to switch it up and see what happened. I had a long commute to work so I had a couple of hours each day to listen, and it was interesting because I found this new music lifted my spirits and I began to feel better. I can honestly say I haven't looked back. I've broadened the music I listen to and have started to find more joy in my life. This isn't because I've acquired anything new except for a new perspective on life. I worked really hard looking for ways to change, desperately trying to steer myself away from suicide.

One day, during that period, I was out for a walk in the woods, and I asked out loud to the universe to show me joy, to teach me what joy is. I declared, "I am open to receiving joy!" I was having a rare moment of exhilaration, and as I walked through the woods alone, I could feel the expansiveness of the nature that surrounded me. I could feel how old the trees were as they towered above me. The ancient Acacia I loved that was so tall and majestic looking, and I could feel the energy they were giving me. I felt happy, I felt free and I wanted to learn.

JOURNALING A JOURNEY

I gave myself permission to start exploring joy again although I still didn't really get it. I thought maybe I'm just not an exuberant kind of person that can put that much energy into my own happiness. I thought there was something wrong with me, and then I made a discovery. Someone told me that joy is not always laughing heartily and throwing our arms up in excitement, joy can also be a feeling of quiet happiness, and a gentle sensation in your heart of elation. Sometimes it is a soft and quiet moment of happiness.

From that day I worked hard to see things differently, and over time I did indeed begin to feel joy flowing toward me, and I realised this was more about gratitude than anything else. My gratefulness for all the different things I had in my life, the people, possessions, experiences. I soon began to feel my spirits lift inside and that gentle elation in my heart rise, or in my solar plexus. When something lifted me inside, I could feel what could only be described as joy but in a quiet and peaceful way. It made me smile, relax, and feel content.

I also found I could laugh in a way I never had before. I laughed with a confidence and freedom and a self-assuredness I'd never had before. I've found that joy can be experienced as a peaceful freedom to be myself in whatever way fits for me, even when it's a quiet moment of calm sitting under the shade of the willow trees I planted four years ago when they were mere twelve-inch sticks in the ground.

Don't get me wrong, I can have a good belly laugh at a comedy show and laugh at jokes just like anyone but when it comes to joy, I feel it as a warm and reassuring sensation in my heart. I feel it as peace in my soul when I know that all is well in my world.

God knows I need joy in my life just now. And sometimes I need to fake it to make it, especially when I'm with my youngest child who needs more reassurance than most about my health. It comes more easily now, like when I stop for a moment and pay attention to my breathing and my surroundings and practice my gratitude for what I have got rather than what I have not got. Right now, there is peace in this moment looking out of my window at the weather, the trees moving in the wild wind, the sound of Rachmaninov being played by my son on the piano rising up from downstairs, and the quiet as I finish writing this piece in the comfort of my own home. Finally, I have found that for me, peace is my joy.

Guided Message

You put so much pressure on yourself dear one to always be the perfect one to have all the answers and know it all when you know so little of this universe and all that it holds. Be still and listen always to your inner heart and your inner child for they are the ones who know what you best need. Be guided by your inner knowing and say, I am at peace, and I trust that all is well. We watch carefully to ensure the opportunities are placed in your path that will serve you best at that time, and when you are following your intuition, you can see them and take the best opportunities available. Your happiness comes not from what you have but from the feeling of what you perceive to have. There are no rules about what happiness should feel like, there is only the moment to live in, and love in, and to enjoy to its fullest. Be enveloped in all that surrounds you as a magical moment and a place of beauty for there is beauty in every creation.

birdlike heart

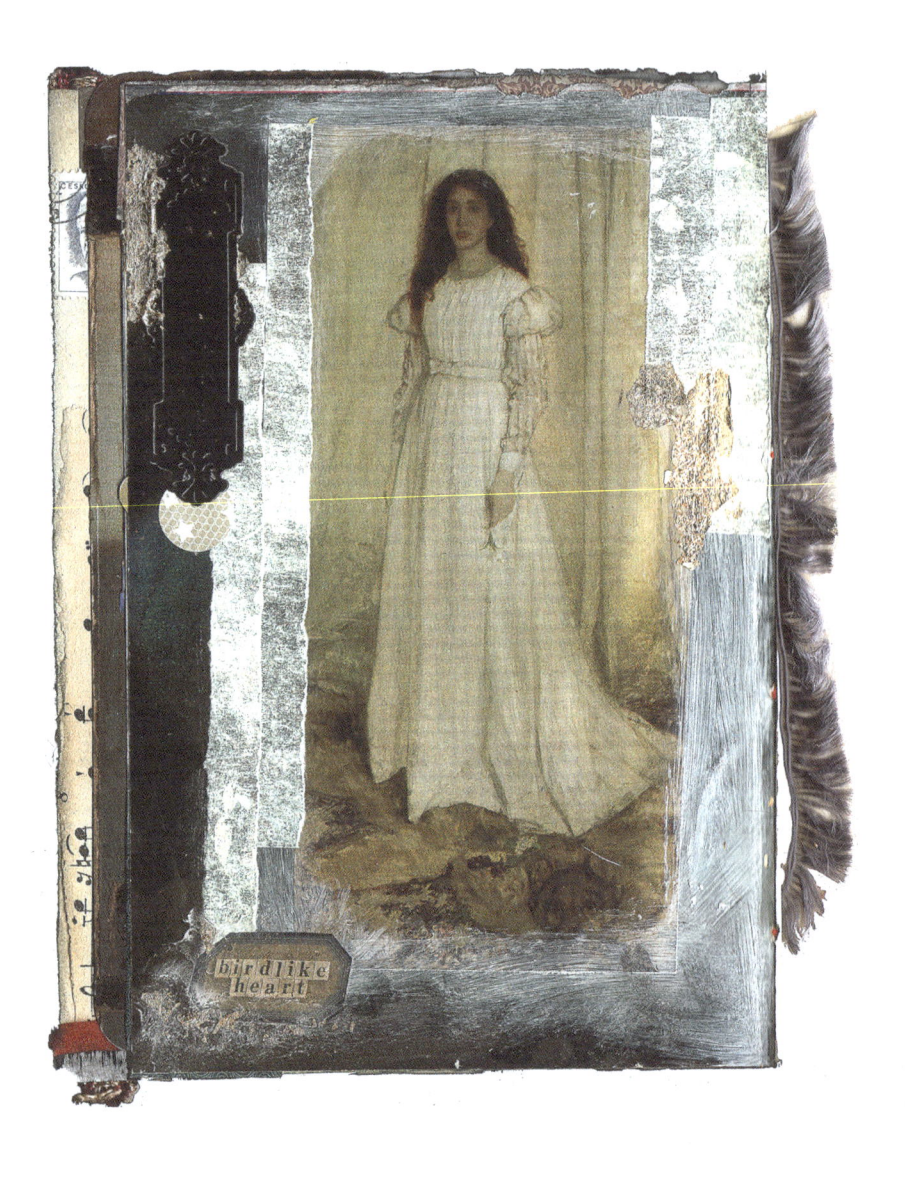

Guardian Angel

Once, I bumped into an old friend I hadn't seen in years whilst walking down the street. He was in an emotional state and needed support. He said I was his guardian angel and he didn't know what he would have done if I hadn't come along in that moment. I didn't do much, just listened to what was happening for him and gave him some time, then we parted company when he was feeling better. But I don't think it was any coincidence I was in the right place at the right time. Sometimes we encounter people in our lives for the briefest of moments, yet they can have the biggest impact.

It was a dark, late October evening. It was cold and I was tired after a long day at work. I had just come off the slip road from the motorway and was heading down the final long stretch of road back home through the rush hour traffic on Great Western Road. I was having one of my lowest days. I was in the middle of some difficult parenting stuff happening at home and I knew it would all kick off when I got in, so I was bracing myself to deal with that.

Layered over that was my sadness. When I was alone it would cover me like a heavy blanket. In some ways it was comforting because it was so familiar, and I had learned how to snuggle into it so well and it fitted just right. I could reach into its corners and draw out a memory to dwell upon and it would snake around me like a tourniquet that I knew could bring relief.

I wished there was some way of ending it all. I was so tired. The kind of tired that sleep doesn't cure or a rest on a warm armchair in a sunny corner. It was the kind of exhaustion that made every move a task, every thought a danger of overloading my batteries and fusing out and it brought with it a desire to not be here anymore. But I had to be here and the part of me that runs the common sense and practical areas of my life just wouldn't let me go. The pain of dragging this despair around with me every day was debilitating. I was brilliant at masking it. Most people who knew me would have had no idea I was feeling that way. There were a few who did, and they were my lifeline when I was drowning.

I slipped into my pattern of morose reflection like most people slip into their comfiest pyjamas, as the traffic came to a halt. I sighed and pulled on the handbrake to wait for it to clear and glanced down the seemingly endless trail of blinking red brake lights ahead of me. The traffic on the other side was at a standstill as well. I'm a people watcher, so I almost always take those opportunities to notice who else is around me and what they're doing. The guy in the car next to me just a few feet away facing the opposite direction was uninteresting to the point that I can't remember anything to describe him with here. But then their lane moved slightly, and the cars shuffled forward one space and he was replaced by a woman. I can't remember what she looked like either which is strange because I will never forget what happened next.

It was like it all happened in slow motion but was over in less than a minute. Her car approached and filled the space left by the previous car. She looked right at me as if she was expecting to see me. As her gaze fell on mine, I had a feeling of transparency. She saw me, I mean really saw me, in a way that no one had ever seen me before. Her eyes locked with mine and in that instant, it was as though she could read my thoughts. Her face turned to concern as she furrowed her brow and mouthed the words, "Are you ok?" I panicked. I knew I was not ok; I was not in the smallest sense of being ok and she knew it. How did she know? A multitude of emotions flooded through me including embarrassment at being seen like that, unmasked and naked. I couldn't handle it. Something about her directness and the clarity with which she seemed to see me was terrifying. I did the only thing I could think of, I put my mask on. I mustered a watery smile and quickly nodded in a brisk and reassuring way, pretending as if I had just been in a daydream.

I could tell by her face she wasn't buying it, and she knew it was a lie. We both knew. She gave me a deep, meaningful look then briefly glanced through her windscreen as her lane slowly started to move. One more fleeting look, and she was gone to be replaced with a line of meaningless cars driving past my window.

My regret was instant, and I wished I hadn't pretended. I wanted to jump out of the car and yell after her to come back and help me somehow. I wanted to fall into her arms and tell her everything. I wanted to bury my head in her shoulder and just cry. But I didn't know how and now she was gone. The moment was gone. I tried to imagine how we could have done it anyway; it was ridiculous. What could she do to help me in the middle of traffic? We couldn't stop everything for her to administer mental health first aid, and yet, if she had stepped out of her car in that moment, I would have been so grateful.

That was six years ago, and I still feel emotional when I think of her, even though I'm all good now and I burned that old blanket a long time ago, but I wonder, I always wonder, what did she see on my face that day that made her stop and connect with me?

I think of her as a guardian angel. Seeing her really shook me up and helped me move a step further along the path to getting some help. She shone a light on how sad and desperate I was feeling and made me realise how bad things had got. Funny how I can't remember what she looked like, and I don't think it was an accident she was there. She was sent to give me a message and I received it well. She may well have saved my life.

Notes

Guided Message

Dear ones, when you are in despair, we are always watching out for you and over you. We send our earth angels to acknowledge and guide you. You are never alone, never on your own. We are always trying to lift you up and see the light and a clear direction.

If you are struggling, then think of us and hold your thoughts in a sacred space. Cradle them as you would a baby and think of yourself as the one to nurture. Too often you forget to nurture and care for yourself. You neglect the most important person in your life, yourself, for without you, you have no life to live! Think of how many people you touch on a daily basis. Think of how many people you are aware of and who come into your presence for your presence, and be conscious of what they and you need, for you are in a constant interaction and dance with each other, playing this game of life and hoping for the best outcomes. Go, and enjoy what this life has to offer and remember to be aware of exactly who you are to each and every person you meet, even when it's for the briefest of moments. You are as loved as you give love.

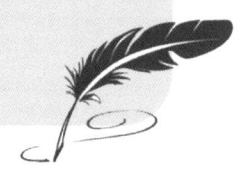

THIS WILL HELP YOU

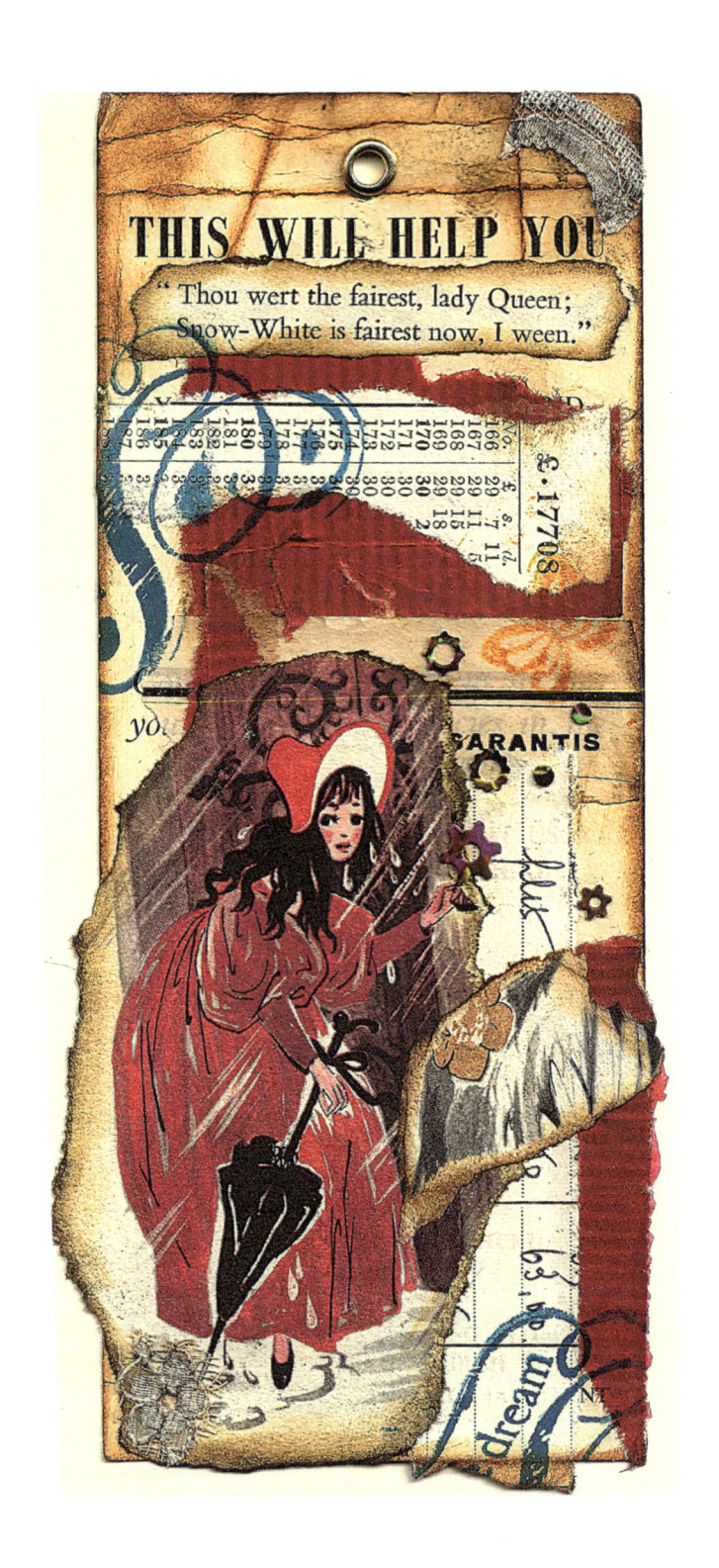

"Thou wert the fairest, lady Queen;
Snow-White is fairest now, I ween."

dream

Ink

When I was a little girl, I remember seeing the Windsor and Newton ink bottle on my mother's writing desk. I don't think I ever saw her use it, but I remember the image from the box with the smiling spider in a top hat creeping across the box weaving his web as he went.

There's always been something wonderful to me about ink, the depth of the colour black, the viscosity and texture of it and the way it could flow from a nib. I often wondered how it was made and was fascinated to learn of different methods of gathering the colour black from things like charcoal and lamp smoke.

My mother used to sit at her writing desk late into the night tapping at her Imperial typewriter, until she upgraded and got a fancy new electric one, and then the tapping got faster. Decades later she gave me the Imperial typewriter and I use it in my art. It had been a gift to her from her father for achieving something, I forget what. I don't know why she gave it to me. We were never close. Ink and typewriters, purveyors of the written word and inky loveliness, the typewriter ribbon rich with ink when it's first placed on the spindles and over time fading with all the words pressed from it onto the paper.

In Primary four we were transitioning from only using pencils to write with and started practicing writing with pens. The teacher, Mrs Ferguson, had asked us to complete a piece of writing using pen and then present it to her for inspection on completion.

I sat at the back of that class, so I had an intimidating distance to walk up to her desk from the back of the long classroom to have her critique of my work. Once I reached her desk, I tentatively held the pages open for her to scrutinise. Two full pages of writing, I was pleased with my work although I can't remember now what I wrote about.

She took the jotter from me, glanced over the writing, and without hesitation she looked over the top rims of her glasses and said, "Wendy, it looks like a spider has dipped its legs in black ink and walked across the page." She then handed my jotter back with a nod to my desk and a raise of her eyebrows, indicating I could now return to my desk, the inference being that I should try again.

JOURNALING A JOURNEY

It was my birthday today, and one of the gifts I received was a bottle of Windsor and Newton black ink with that same image of the spider on the box and the memory came back to me as it has done before, and I wondered, did my teacher have a bottle of the same ink at her writing desk, and is that how she arrived at that metaphor? Resting my head back on my pillow this memory drifts in and back out of my mind and I'm considering what I'm going to do with this delicious, fresh bottle of ink.

Using a dipping pen, I'll explore making marks as well as trying my hand at writing beautifully and creatively. To be honest, I don't think my handwriting will ever be called beautiful, that spirited spider never seems to have left my side, but I will lean into the flow of ink and words to see what occurs, and if it looks like a spider has walked across the page, then I'll still be happy with that.

Notes

Guided Message

How joyful to find the humour in one's imperfections, and in amongst the power of the written word. Even more important to acknowledge that your writing may not always be perfect either in form or script and yet it is still always relevant in some way. Do not underestimate that power and practice it often as a way to express how you feel, to yourself in private, and others publicly. There is strength and courage in doing both. Using whatever means is available is important too. Do not get tangled up in what is right or wrong in what tools you should use, they are all adequate and as long as they serve their purpose then it is correct. Too often you allow yourself to be caught up in methods rather than the simplicity of getting to the point of the written and expressed word. Humour too, is one of your greatest tools in writing as that is one of the easiest ways to reach an audience and one must work on cultivating that. We thank you for sharing your words with the world!

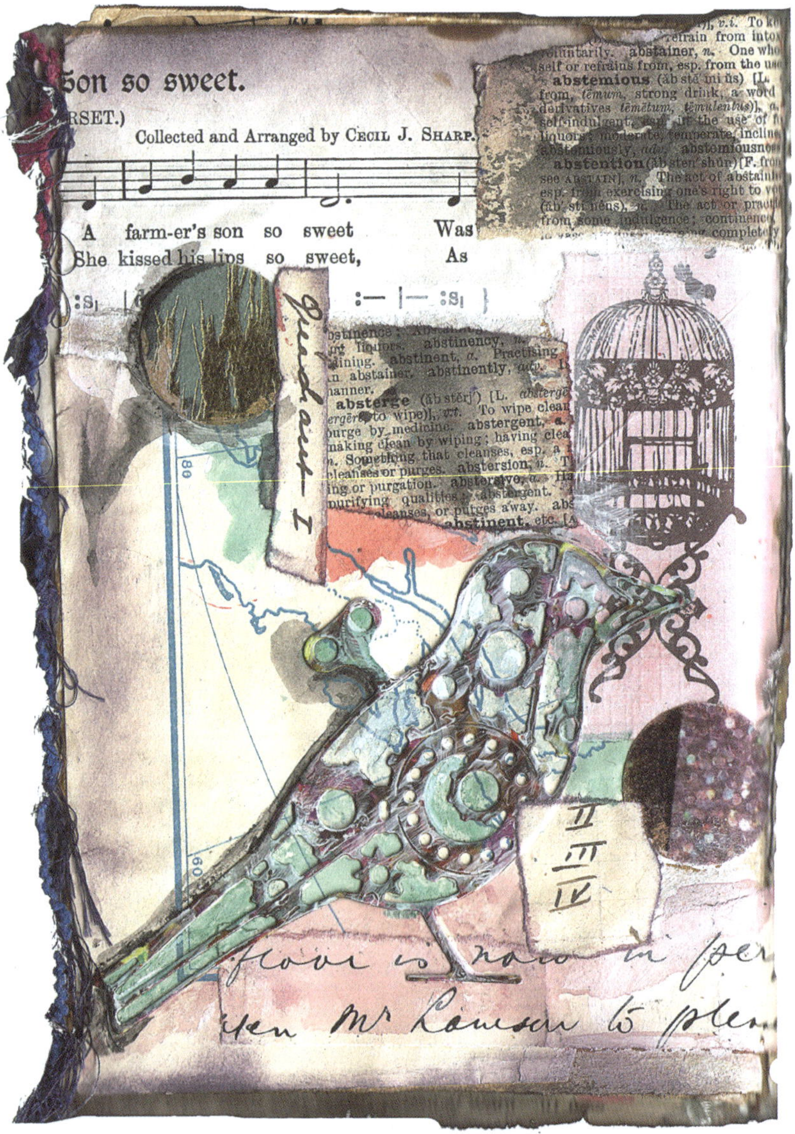
Son so sweet.
RSET.)
Collected and Arranged by Cecil J. Sharp.
A farm-er's son so sweet Was
She kissed his lips so sweet, As
abstainer, n. One who
self or refrains from, esp. from the use
abstemious
abstention
abstinency
abstinent, a. Practising
abstinently
absterge
To wipe clean
abstergent
abstersion, n.
abstersive, a.
abstinent.

Liminal Limbo

I've never really looked at my own death in the eye like this before. For many years I thought I wanted to die but what I didn't know or realise at the time, was that I was in control of that thought and desire, and therefore it was easy to be fearless. I fantasised often about killing myself, how, and when I would do it and what the aftermath would look like. It was narcissistic behaviour at times but also, a lot of the time I was just feeling desperate and lost with no solutions to hand for all the problems I felt I had. It was excruciating and went on for too many years.

Standing at the other side of all of that with my suicidal thoughts processed and all my demons exorcised, I have a clean slate. I am at peace. I have a life that I'm in love with and grateful for. So, when the prospect of death rears its beguiling head back into my life again, it is different. It's not on my terms anymore, and it's really scary. I'm not scared of dying, in and of itself, I have a strong spiritual practice that supports me in a knowing that when I die, I will be returned to source in the most gentle and beautiful way, and I will be happy with the life I've had. I have no regrets in this life, except for not having gone to see Queen perform in 1985 when I was fourteen at Milton Keynes and instead going on holiday to Benidorm with a friend. It was a great holiday, but I should have seen Queen; Freddie Mercury had been my hero since I was seven years old, and the opportunity never came up again.

It's not easy to look death in the eye and have a conversation with his good self and play that game of chess at the edge of time. Now, I am older I know what loss is, and what I must lose. Now, just as my life got really fricking good, I am presented with the very thing I spent many years plotting and praying for. And why didn't I do it if I wanted it that badly? I hear some of you ask. It always came back to a deep inner knowing that I could get through my struggles and that there were powerful lessons to be learnt in them. I wasn't wrong in thinking that either, I learnt a great deal from all my hardships, and they've been put to good use in the work that I do.

I'm standing with barely one step over the threshold of my second half-century, staring down the barrel of a gun, and death is still not an option and for even more reasons than before. I have too much to give. So much love left to give for a family I do not want to leave, with children I haven't finished bringing up, and amazing, loving friendships. I've made too many plans for work and creative projects, with even in the last couple of months people contacting me, interested in knowing more about my work, and I'm so eager to share and collaborate. I'm not done yet; It feels like I just got started.

   I'm guessing I'm not alone in my experience of being in the dance of liminal limbo; at the beginning of a cancer diagnosis but not yet having seen the oncologist to understand more about what type it is and the plan for treatment, how long it will be and what options are potentially available to me. Facing the dancers pole held low by my surgeon and pain management nurse, wondering how the hell I'm going to make it through as the music plays on. I'll keep on absorbing the inordinate amount of love and support that has come pouring out to me and my family and be grateful for all of that and all that I have. One day at a time, one foot in front of the other, knowing that I can still help others in some way, even if it's just sharing this experience.

Notes

Guided Message

Your capacity for hope and the gathering of other souls within that hope is beyond what our expectations would be. We want to see you heal in whatever form that takes and within that process we see you make the best of a difficult situation. You are indeed surrounded by people who love you, and so many more than you realise. They come lining up to thank you for your service to them, even at times when you didn't know you were helping someone with just a smile or a small gesture. You have more capacity for kindness than most and when you see that, it makes your life a little easier as you then feel more deserving of the help you need. Acceptance is at the core of this diagnosis and the vision to see it through to the end, which you will. You are at a turning point in your life and are rounding a corner that has been long approaching. Take your time to navigate it fully and explore all its alleys as there are experiences to be had within this particular experience that you cannot have elsewhere. Do not be afraid of what lies ahead and instead embrace all the nuances and places you will go. As always, you will make the best of it and ensure that it is shared with those who need it. All power to you and this journey.

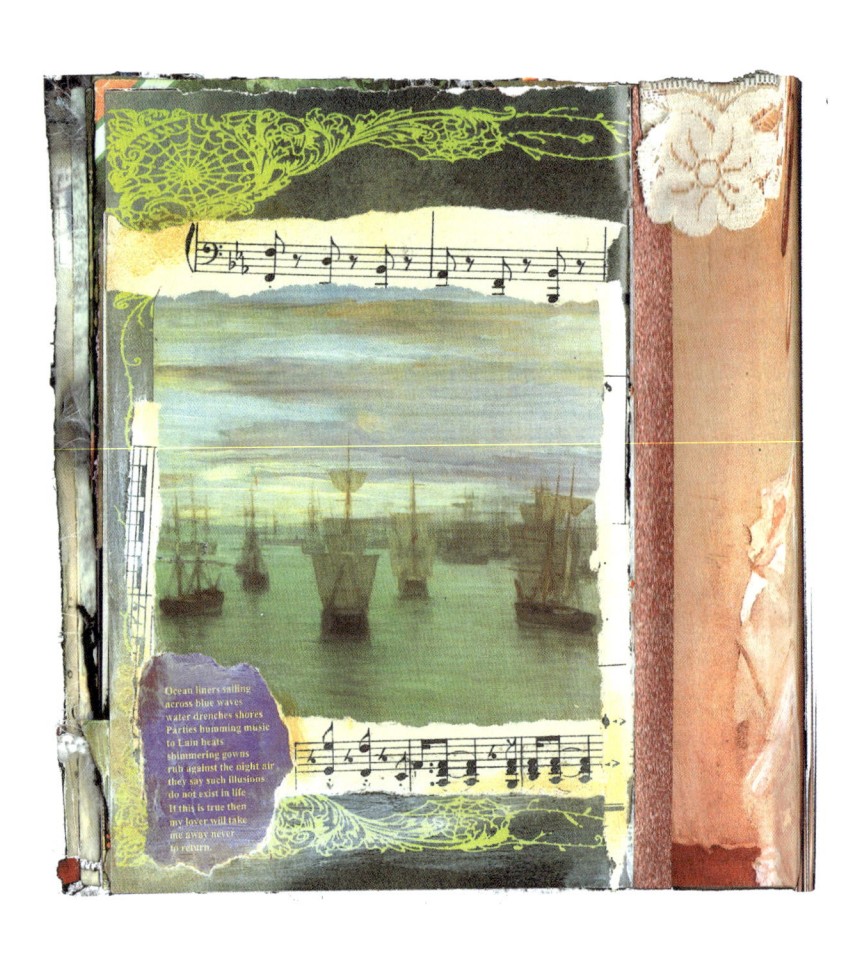

Ocean liners sailing
across blue waves
water drenches shores
Parties humming music
to Latin beats
shimmering gowns
rub against the night air
they say such illusions
do not exist in life
If this is true then
my lover will take
me away never
to return.

Open Up

There can be a lot of fear and misunderstanding surrounding counselling and therapy. I've spoken to many people who are afraid to get help because they think they will have to share every little detail about their lives, and that's not the case. Here, I will talk about it from my perspective with a little of what I've learned. Although don't take my word alone for it, do your own research and ask other people what it was like for them. Anyway, I'll briefly tell you about the different experiences I had and where I ended up.

When I was twenty-eight, I had my first mental break; I was in a bad way and I knew I needed to see a therapist, and fast. I didn't know how to find a good one, so I opened the yellow pages, as this was before the internet had properly developed, so we still used phone books to find each other. I flipped it open at the therapist/counsellor section and stuck my finger on the first one I saw, and I phoned them. As it transpired, he was a hypnotherapist, and he was quite good, but I didn't get into anything deep with him and I couldn't open up, I just wasn't ready. However, I did take away a key learning from him; that I could question my beliefs, and that has continued to serve me very well to this day.

What this meant for me was that he gave me 'permission' to look at all the things I had been told were true and ask myself if that was the case. I had been brought up with rigid thinking and ideals that I did not like so this was the beginning of disentangling myself from that sticky web. Most importantly, he guided me back on track again so I could carry on with everyday life, returning to stability and my job.

The second time I saw a counsellor I was thirty-eight, and this was a year after my first son was born. Looking back, I clearly had post-partum depression as well as whatever else was going on for me. I went to a well-known counselling centre and had about ten sessions courtesy of the NHS. I talked about all the things that I thought were causing my problems but by the end I felt like I hadn't made much progress and was still as depressed as before. They couldn't offer me any more sessions and so it was left at that. It had been productive in that I had the chance to air some real issues to someone who didn't know me and have them validated, but he was unable to move me past it.

Finally, I hit rock bottom, a real low where I crashed so hard I could barely get up again. I'd pushed it all too far and I could no longer cope with even the basics. This was just six years ago at forty-six, and again I self-referred to the same counselling centre who, after ten sessions, then referred me on to a trauma specialist where I was diagnosed with Complex Post Traumatic Stress Disorder (CPTSD). I'm grateful to that counsellor as she recognised that she was not the right person to support me and that my problems ran deeper, and therefore referring me on was the right thing to do. I was fortunate to receive this support on the NHS and it lasted for three and a half years.

You see, there's only so much your brain can take before it just goes into overload. I don't think this is something that just applies to me, our minds can only cope with so much before they start to protest and demand some proper attention. I had always self-diagnosed and believed I knew what was wrong with me, and up to a point I did. But that's not how it works. We need an objective viewpoint, someone else to help us look at things from a different direction or perspective. My therapist was amazing and I'm going to outline why so if you're looking for a therapist it might work as a guideline for good practice, something I hadn't fully experienced until that point. This is just my opinion, so take from it what you will.

For the first nine months she focused primarily on my self-care, this was due to the trauma I had experienced and the mindset I had developed, I really didn't know how to look after myself and tended to prioritise others over me. I came very low down on the list of things that were important, and that was not good for my mental or physical health, and that's not good for healthy parenting either.

As we approached the nine months mark my ability to recognise my own self-worth had increased and opened up my mind, and I started to have flashbacks and remember things I never knew had happened. It was very disturbing. This was a huge turning point for me and one that my therapist navigated with great care. I was a mess and deeply traumatised and triggered. I barely knew how to function at times. Interestingly, my job helped me stay afloat at that point for a few months, as the routine of work was useful, and then I took some sick leave when I got too overwhelmed. What was important during those months of early disclosure was that my therapist was extremely careful not to put words into my mouth or make any suggestions or allusions to anything that may or may not have happened to me. This was necessary, as I had so few memories, I had a hard time believing any of it was true and that I had made it all up. However, she was able to piece it all together and make sense of it for me which was crucial. This does not mean she made up a story from what I told her, it means that as an objective, professional listener she could see more clearly what had happened from the evidence that I gave to her in different ways including dates and locations etc. This proved to be critical as I improved and started to look back on it all and I could clearly see it was all my own narrative and fully authentic. For someone with few concrete memories that was essential.

It was a profoundly hard time, but she held an objective and compassionate space. She never crossed boundaries or tried to be my friend, something I've experienced and seen from other counsellors. She could draw me out when I became too internalised and empathised in a way that made me feel genuinely heard and validated. She was completely authentic in her approach and never tried to be something or someone else. She respected my wishes and worked hard to help me recover and I will be eternally grateful to her for all of that.

She held that space for me so beautifully and walked me towards a gentle ending ensuring I had covered everything I needed to. There was no stone left unturned, and I knew I could ask her anything and be completely honest. I told her things that no-one else knows and I will take to my grave. I had, and still do have, absolute trust in her. When I saw her for the last time, I was ready to leave. I left with a feeling of freedom and happiness that I never knew was possible.

During therapy I learnt how to laugh again. I learnt what peace meant. I became a different person, and it opened me up to a whole new world of possibilities. I learnt how to live again, instead of just existing from one day to the next, always ruminating and drifting in and out of the trauma responses of fight, flight and most often freeze. I live a completely different life inside my head now and it's a place of peace and absolute freedom. I have renewed confidence and high self-esteem. I even experience a gentle joy, something that had always eluded and confused me.

I could say much more but I hope this brief account is of some help to anyone who may be looking for support. Talking therapy isn't for everyone, especially for young people as they are usually still too close to the time when the trauma happened. Often, we need some distance before we are ready to process, and there are different levels of processing as I think I've illustrated here. I was not ready to do the deep therapy work in my twenties or thirties.

Therapy takes time and a lot of patience. It can be hard work, and at times I wanted to give up, but it was worth sticking in, and I don't think it's an exaggeration to say that it saved my life.

Notes

Guided Message

The sharing of experiences is vital for learning and understanding how to grow and for relationships to build. We are delighted to see this subject being discussed as there is indeed a great deal of fear around talking about the things that have happened in people's lives that were not good at all. This is at the heart of the problem, and your willingness to be open about your own experience will be helpful for others. Learn to open up more and be fearless in sharing your experiences. You only have this one chance to do it, to make it right, and help to heal this world, and every time you do it makes a difference. Do not be afraid to be honest as without that we have nothing. Take heart that when you speak your truth there is always someone who is eager to hear it.

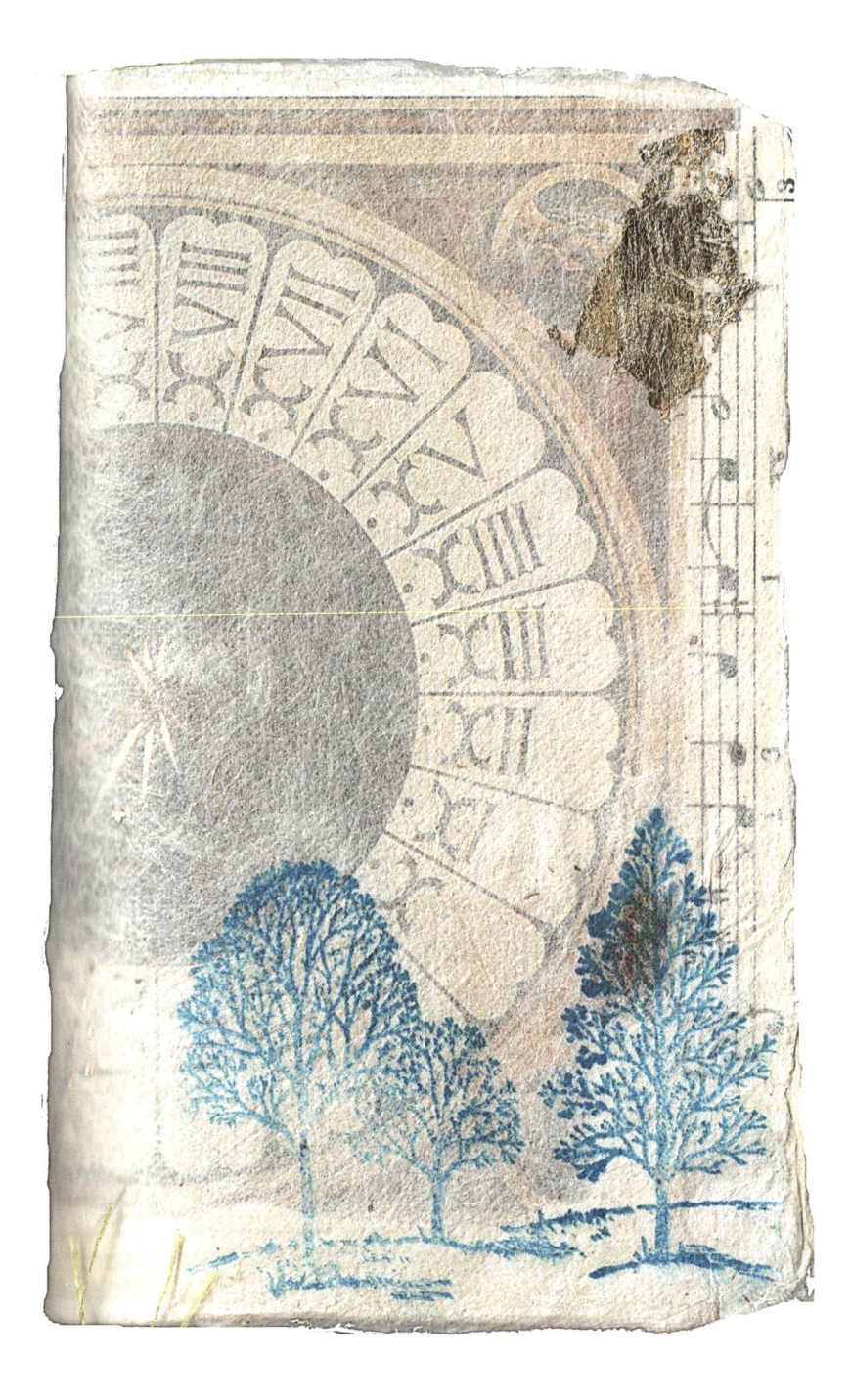

The Diagnosis

When I sat down in the surgeons' office for the results of my biopsy, I had convinced myself he was going to tell me he could remove the tumour from the cavity behind my eye. I had created a story that had me going in for the surgery to remove it, and then the pressure in my head would begin to reduce and therefore so would all my symptoms. Within a few weeks my pain would lessen, and I would start the process of coming off all the drugs I was on. The result being that I would be back at work, and life by February at the latest and I could put all of this behind me. I don't know why I had decided that this was the outcome, except that I guess it was the best-case scenario and that's what I was hoping for, naturally.

The month before, I had seen a psychic medium, something I had never previously done. It was just something that came up and felt right, so I contacted her for a reading, and we met online. One of the things she said about my health, was that treatment would be quick. She had been very reassuring and told me that the best team was being put together for me and

THE DIAGNOSIS

ultimately the outcome was good. However, she also said that it was good that I already had short hair when she was referring to the treatment, and we both laughed at that. I knew what was being intimated by it, that when people receive chemotherapy, they often lose their hair, I allowed it to go over my head and blanked out that scenario, instead focusing on what else she was saying, like about it being quick, which fitted in well with my surgery scenario. Funny how we do that, isn't it? We like to rearrange information to fit our preferred narrative. It's called confirmation bias, and in that moment, the last thing I wanted was to be told that my comfortable little story was not going to come true, even though she said there would be a happy ending by taking the other path.

That's one of the things about me, I always like to take the path less travelled, and all my life have tended to swim against the tide when everyone else is going with it. Although I also do believe in going with the flow and not fighting what's in front of me, following the signs as they come up and being easy going in my life, whilst at the same time doing my best not to be typical, not to fit in too well, be slightly different, and not follow the crowd. I do this not to be difficult but so I always look for the most interesting corners of life, to avoid falling into the trap of boredom and sameness and getting into a rut, and most importantly, to have a life of art and creativity in as many different ways as is possible. This way of thinking comes from an innate distrust of authority, born from a childhood of gaslighting and never being able to trust the authorities in my life and always being the butt of the joke, which led to the first part of my life being about conformity and never doing what I wanted to do. Instead, I work to keep one step ahead of anything that could get in the way of achieving my dreams, I keep my cards close to my chest, and research to ensure an element of caution and to protect myself.

Unfortunately, on this occasion, there was nothing to research and all I could do was wait for the results of the biopsy, and in the interim make up a story that fitted my preferred narrative, completely ignoring the possibility of other scenarios.

So, when the niceties had passed with the hello's and I'd told him how I'd been feeling the last three weeks and how my pain medication had been working, I was utterly crushed when he told me firstly, that it was not benign and secondly, that surgery was not possible due to too many risks. It was an atypical tumour, and the irony was not lost on me.

He scooted over to me on his wheeled stool and put a comforting hand on my shoulder as I began to crumble and cry. I just could not believe what I was hearing. How did this happen to me? I immediately thought of

THE DIAGNOSIS

my boys and wondered how was I going to tell them? How to tell my mother and father-in-law who had given us a lift to the hospital and were waiting to take us home again? Suddenly my whole life crashed around my shoulders and a hundred questions burst from my head, the splinters and shards from the edifice that had just shattered all around me.

I had always been against chemotherapy, I balked at the thought of putting all those chemicals directly into my bloodstream, flooding me with their poison but as he began to describe the treatment and how it would work, there was a feeling deep inside me that knew this was the only way to go. And I held onto my lifeline, the man whose patience, and strength seemed to be endless. The warmth of my husband's hand, my anchor in this sea of pain and uncertainty.

And maybe my hair would fall out, but I really didn't care about that. I only cared that I could get well and continue with this life that, once upon a time, I didn't think I wanted to have.

Guided Message

You are cloaked with strategies to protect yourself and now find yourself adrift in an ocean of possibilities that have never been considered before. This is where your great strength comes in and you begin to involve and call upon your higher power for support and guidance, and that is exactly what we are here for.

No-one should travel this journey alone, least of all when it becomes as hard as this. We are always here to support and help and you need only ask when you need our guidance. We will never refuse and will always find a way to tell you what to do. Be silent and listen, for we are whispering in your ear the answers to your questions, and you will intuitively know what you must do.

Do not worry dear one for we have got your back. In terms of treatment, again you must follow your inner guidance as well as take good advice from professionals. There are merits to both systems, and it is not impossible to combine the two.

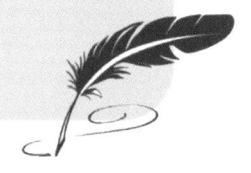

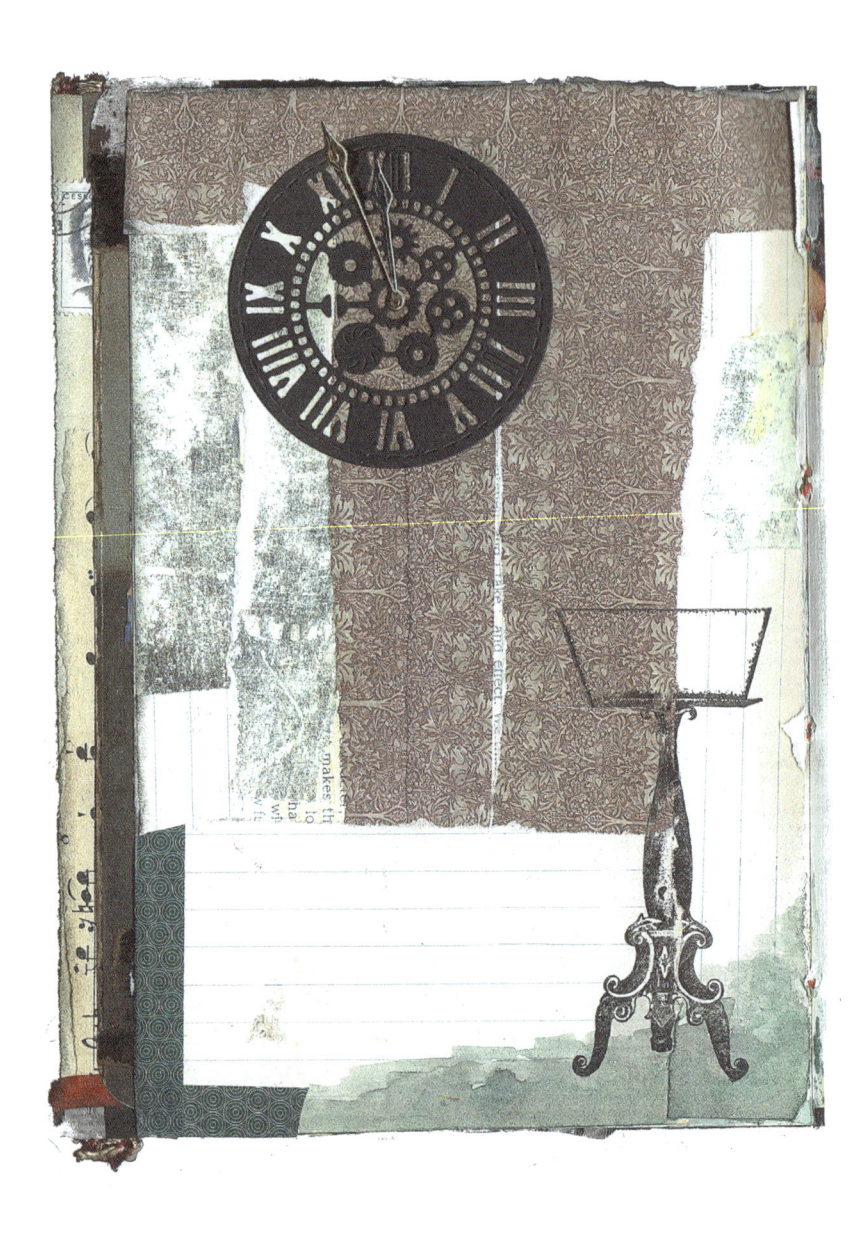

The Piano

There was a time when I could be reduced to tears just by hearing someone play the piano, say at a party or an event or one of those ones they sometimes leave in train stations. I would be stopped in my tracks at the sound of it and often just have to leave the room or walk away, the strength of emotion it awoke in me was too much to bear. I didn't understand where it came from for a long time. For example, I remember once being at a wedding and sobbing in a room listening to the sounds of the piano being played elsewhere, and being at a complete loss as to why I was so destroyed just by hearing it. The pain in my heart felt so deep, the sadness so profound. I was trapped in freeze mode, and it took some time to gather myself back together into some semblance of coping to join the guests again.

My son started playing the piano when he was ten years old, and I wasn't prepared for the onslaught of emotion and memory that it would bring.

When I was growing up my eldest brother played the piano. I think he must have enjoyed it as it seemed to

THE PIANO

me like he played almost every night for hours. I loved the sound of him playing the piano, he was good, and it was comforting. I particularly remember when he was learning how to play Beethoven's Moonlight Sonata. It was a dreamy and evocative piece and I never tired of listening to it. Now and again, I would sit beside him on the piano stool and watch him, I loved being near him, my big brother. I looked up to him and admired him. I tried to emulate him and took an interest in the things he was interested in, so his favourite bands became mine, Deep Purple, Queen, and The Eagles.

I would sneak into his room when he wasn't there and steal his books to read, All Quiet on the Western Front and The Hobbit. He never got his copy of The Hobbit back, even though it had been given to him by our grandma and signed with a loving message for his birthday. I confessed to him thirty years later and he let me keep it. But the piano, it brought a warmth to the house and was comforting, it cut through silence, harsh words, the cold, and it stirred my imagination.

Hearing the piano in my own home decades later was a huge surprise as it came out of nowhere. There had been no indication that either of my children would want to play the piano, and we didn't even have one in our flat at the time. I mean, I loved it, I just never expected the reel of emotions that it brought up. He would play Chopin, and I was compelled to stop what I was doing and would become transfixed. I froze and was transported to a time when I was not happy at all, and yet the piano was a happy moment within that turmoil. The confusion was great, and I often had to hide my tears as a well of emotion rose up inside me with no explanation. When he eventually learnt how to play Moonlight Sonata it was like a tsunami, and I didn't know what to do with myself.

When I was fifteen, I wanted to kill myself. It was not the first time I felt that way. One night I went to our bathroom, I took out some paracetamol and I started to swallow them. I got to five and I stopped. I'm really not sure why but I did, and then I went downstairs to my brother who was, as usual, playing the piano. I sat next to him on the stool, and I told him I needed to talk to him. I had never talked to him in this way before, neither him nor my other brothers. None of us talked to each other ever, there was little to no emotional connection built between any of us. He stopped playing the piano and turned to listen to me. I told him I had just taken too many paracetamols but not enough to kill myself, but I told him that was what I wanted to do. Then I started to spill about how I was feeling, and a lot of emotion began to tumble out, and he sat there not knowing what to do with it all.

  I don't know how long we sat there with me talking but suddenly my mum stormed in like a volcano erupting, and demanded to know what was going on. She had been listening at the door to our conversation and started ranting about how ungrateful I was and how she had given me everything: food, clothes, a lovely house, and I cried and tried to explain to her how I was feeling.

  I tried to deflect it away from her even though she was the root cause of it all and instead just explained how bad I was feeling and that I wanted help. We were both crying, and our voices got louder and louder, and quickly we were screaming at each other until it reached a crescendo which is how all our arguments ended up. Eventually it stopped because I got a nosebleed.

  I always got a nosebleed when I got too upset. These were no ordinary nosebleeds, they could last for up to an hour with a strong, steady flow of blood. This was usually how things ended, and with the issue at hand left completely unresolved.

  And there I was listening to my son play the piano and I'm crumbling away inside with every note played, sinking farther into the past. It seems like the light has dimmed and I'm watching him play as if from outside of my body and I'm not really present in the room. I want him to stop, and I also want him to play endlessly. The bittersweetness of being trapped in a moment from the past where I am safe and yet unsafe. I know everything and yet I know nothing. It is a place of limbo and purgatory where I can tell my younger self what she should do and I can see all sides of the story, even if I don't want to.

Eventually, I took the story to my therapist who helped me to unpick and unravel all the threads and reweave them into a new story, one where I could see the beauty of my child playing without me drifting away and instead experience the pleasure of being in the moment, witnessing his talent and the joy of him playing without melancholy or sadness rising from the past.

Now and again, I will visit that old childhood piano stool and remember this story, not so much with sadness but rather to sit in companionship with it, and know that none of it is real now, and instead see that the piano now brings me a pleasure and happiness I never thought possible, and that is a real gift.

Notes

Guided Message

Dear child you see so clearly what has arisen and how you have healed from your past traumas. Even though they can still bring you sadness you are able to sit in the present moment with your stories and not disappear into a dimension that in reality no longer exists. You are here now and living your life in the best way you can manage and that too is a real gift. Bring this gift to others with your presence of mind, and your wisdom, which is drawn from these past experiences. You are a fount of knowledge in many ways and are one who finds it possible to weave past and present together not only for yourself but for others too. Do not be shy about sharing this skill as it helps many. Continue this healing journey as it is indeed an endless one within this realm, and a privilege for us to behold it happening as you make such a good job of it. Remember you are loved through all these times past and present and that we are always here for you.

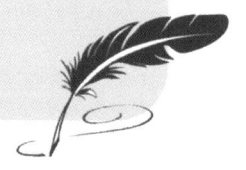

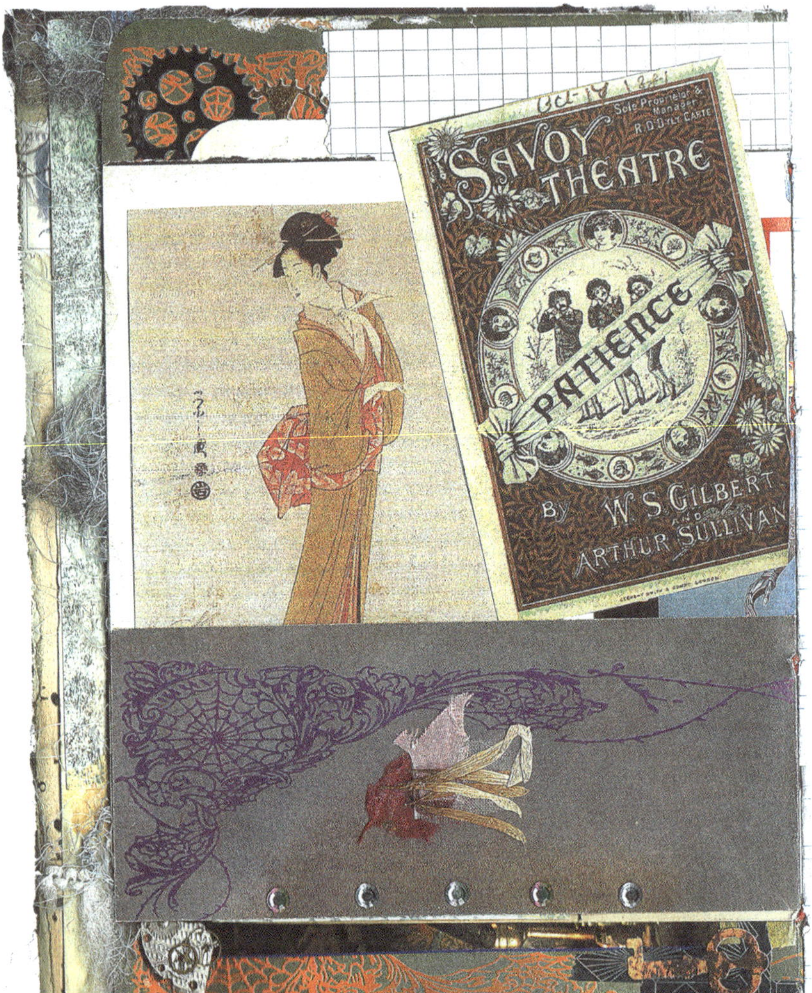
SAVOY THEATRE
PATIENCE
By W. S. GILBERT AND ARTHUR SULLIVAN

Pain

I'm having a bad pain day, so I'll share my experience of pain. I don't have pain like this every day, and it doesn't happen too often thankfully, although I've had more days like this recently.

The whole of the right side of my head is numb and the pain is focused on my eye and nose as that's where the tumour is. It's sharp, it's tingling, it's numb, did I say sharp? It's like needles stabbing at precise places that make me jump. There's a dull throb and ache and it travels up and down my face. One side of my mouth and tongue is numb so I fluff my words a lot and I've been stammering a bit lately, I'm not sure why, maybe that's tiredness, maybe it's the increase in morphine or inflammation from the immunotherapy. Brushing my teeth feels weird because I can't feel them on that side. At times, the pain breaks across my skull like a blazing light, a huge wave of broken glass crashing against the barrier of my mind, and for a moment I'm blinded. The image of bright crystals glittering in a dim light comes into my head as I feel the spasm.

I try to relax and take my attention off it but it doesn't work for long.

PAIN

And I'm tired. A heavy lidded, can't keep my eyes open, kind of tired. As I'm typing I drift off into a mild doze until my husband comes in with a cup of tea, and I wake up again and notice that I dozed off mid-sentence. That'll be the 120mg of morphine I took an hour and a half ago starting to kick in, and hopefully it'll start doing its job of killing off the pain soon. I've been taking my breakthrough pain meds all day but it's stubborn today, refusing to move. Typing is slow and tedious, one letter at a time, then stop, or a whole sentence, then doze off. If I close my eyes for one second I fall asleep.

I feel the pain in my ear creeping down my neck to the lymph gland where there's a cheeky wee bit of 5mm cancer which I wish would just go away so we can keep it nice and simple; all in the head. Huh, that's what they used to say when I was young if we got into one of our fights, "It's all in your head, you're mad, you belong in an asylum!" Oh, dozed off again there, you've got to laugh really, it's ridiculous. I wake with a start when I hear my son shout from his bedroom next door while he's gaming.

I wear glasses now as I explain elsewhere in the book. It hurts to wear them on a day like today. Having anything touch my face feels excruciating and they rest on the exact pain point that's the worst, the bridge of my nose. So, I sit watching programmes or reading books whilst holding them an inch or so off my face so I can still see but they're not touching my face. There's nothing I can do while I'm typing. I think it's amazing that even when in pain I can fall asleep. That happens at bedtime too when I have to do my best to relax and make sleep happen. In these daytime moments, trying to wake up is like swimming through water in a dream. I'm caught in a riptide and it's pulling me relentlessly back out to sea; down and under. The strength of the pull is compelling and hard to ignore, and from somewhere under this expanse I can hear the TV in the distance. I try hard to emerge, and it feels like an age before I'm able to surface again.

It'll soon be bedtime and if previous days are anything to go by, I should start coming right just as it's time to go to sleep, which is good because at least I won't be in pain during the night. But it gets to bedtime and there's no sign of it changing. I take another two doses of my breakthrough pain med and pray that it works. When it gets this bad I start praying to my higher power and asking for help. I should probably have started praying sooner but I always forget. The pain makes me forget everything when it overwhelms me, and anything sensible that I would use to help myself just flies out the window.

When I say praying, it's not a religious thing, it's more like meditating and placing my attention on something more positive. I believe we have a higher power and source that is always looking out for us and is waiting to help in any way it can. I find by doing this it can help calm me down and clear my mind enough to think about what the next best thing I can do will be. I have a number of meditations I've found online that I can listen to as well. However, lately the weather has been wild, wet, and windy, and I love the sound of the rain drumming on the kitchen roof below the bedroom window, the wind howling through the trees and rattling the slate tiles on the roof. I find it soothing to listen to, and it can help me fall asleep. Once again I come back to nature as a way of soothing what ails me. Succour for the soul no matter whether its good weather or bad, or if I'm feeling good or bad. And who's to say what is good or bad anyway? As the Scottish comedian Billy Connolly says, "There's no such thing as bad weather, just the wrong clothes." Well, I'll take a walk in wild, wet weather over pain any day, and since I can't go for a walk, then I shall listen to it instead.

Guided Message

Once more you are sharing the hardest parts of your life for others to hear and that's no bad thing because they can relate to them, or at least some of them can. For those who cannot relate then it is good for them to hear to develop and understand compassion for those who experience this. It is not easy to share and equally it is not easy to hear but no matter, it is what it is and that is what is important. Always be your own person and do not shape yourself into what you think others need you to be. Remain true to yourself and who you are. You will never please everyone and you are not meant to. You will offend some people and that is also ok. You are here to share love, you are here to model compassion, you are here for love, you are here to be who you are. You all are.

No matter how much pain you are in you can still have compassion, that is our message. Pain can change you, either in a positive way or a negative way, it is up to you to choose which it will be. The youngest of our children on this planet need compassion more than anything in order to grow a new world that is filled with it. Let your hearts open to the possibilities of love and pain living side by side.

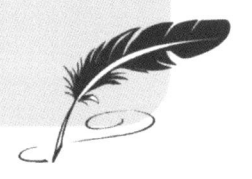

Smooth me, I'll be your friend.

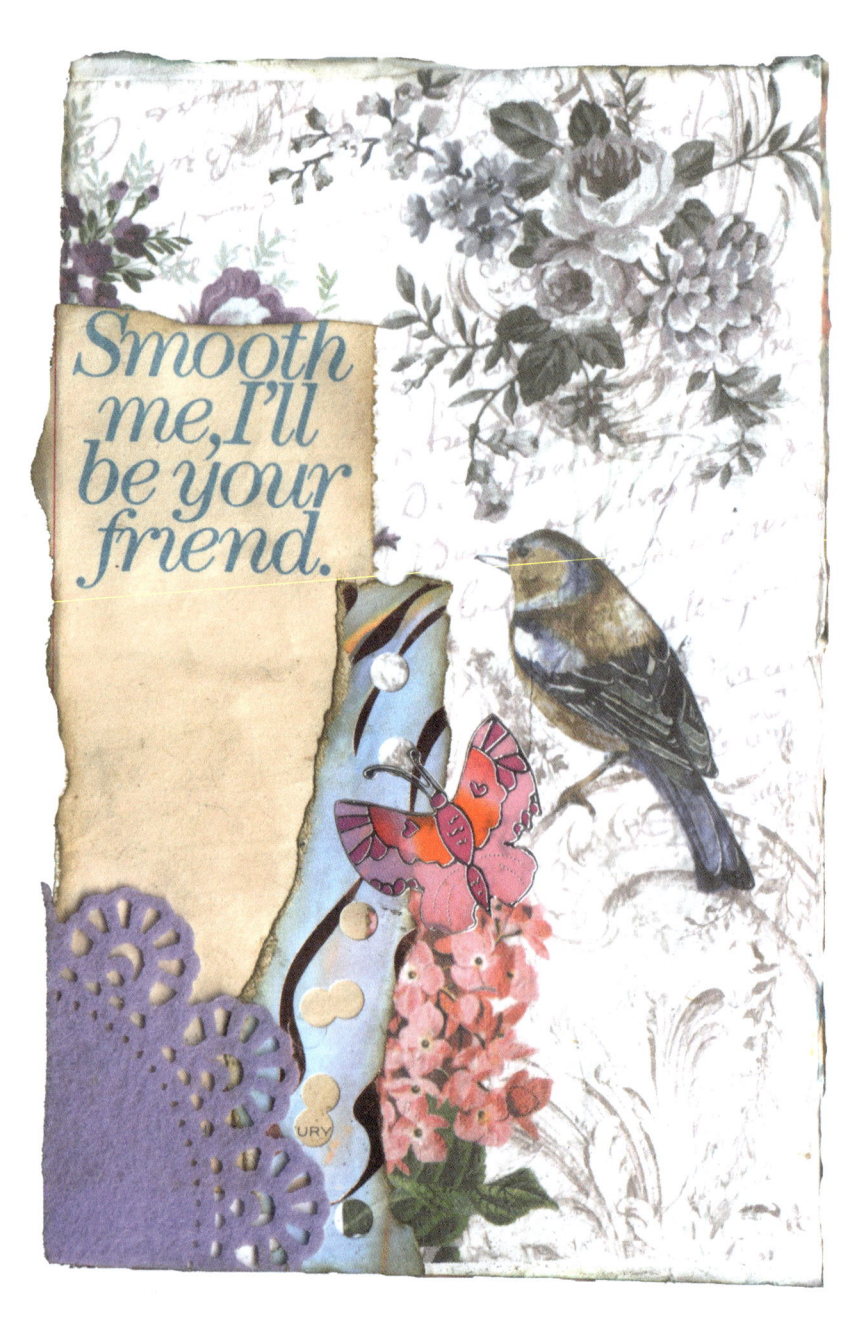

The System of Love

The first time I said the word love in the context of an emotion, and not just talking about how much I loved my new jacket or a friends' hairdo, was with my first boyfriend. I really did love him, and although I was unpractised in using the word, I knew it was the real thing. It felt slightly embarrassing at first, forming the words in my mouth and saying them out loud but it felt nice. It felt good to be in a romantic and loving relationship and feel that love returned, for the first time. I was eighteen. Eighteen years without ever being told I was loved. I think that's really sad.

When I was growing up the word 'love' was never used. I was never told that someone loved me. I never heard anyone say the words 'I love you'. It only became weird as I got older and I noticed that other people said it, like if I was at a friends' house and their parent said it to my friend, and I would feel a bit awkward but not quite know why.

In the seventies, there was this cute cartoon in the papers, it was called 'Love Is…' and it featured a naked,

THE SYSTEM OF LOVE

but sexless looking boy and girl who would model what different types of love could be such as, 'Love is… reading a book together' showing the couple snuggled on a love seat reading a book, or 'Love is… someone to scratch the itch you can't reach' with one of them scratching the back of the other. I really enjoyed these cartoons and bought the sticker album, and each week bought a packet of the collector stickers to put in it. I collected them all, but the album went missing, and I lost it forever, something I still lament to this day. Love always felt important, and yet elusive to me. I didn't know what it was meant to feel like or look like.

I was always one for using cliches like, 'love makes the world go round' and 'all you need is love' but you see, I believed they were true even when people laughed at me for my idealistic nature. I still do believe in those cliches and everything I do comes from a place of love, but it's got me into some amount of trouble, I was far too naïve when I was younger and had no understanding of boundaries and how to keep myself safe. So, in what felt like an endless search for true love and a partner that would love me for who I am, I got into a lot of trouble, some of it serious.

When we don't teach our children how to love it leaves a huge gap in their life lessons and learning.

JOURNALING A JOURNEY

Love is a fundamental resource in our lives; don't we all live for it? Almost every song written is about love. Thousands of poems and stories are written on the theme of love, and I think it's because we are born to love. We are born to be here on this earth to love and to make it as beautiful a place as possible in every way, and love can do that. When we do something that comes from a place of love we create beauty. We see that most obviously in art and music but there are other places where that can happen too, such as governmental systems changing things at a practical level.

Here in Scotland the idea of love is the cornerstone of Scotland's commitment to young people with experience of being in care, it's called The Promise, an aspirational document outlining a system for making support and services better and more empathic and understanding of their specific needs, thus providing them with better chances in life to ensure "they will grow up loved, safe, and respected". This is supported by all the Scottish Parliament's political parties. People are working hard to change institutional systems to start operating on a new level, and this is illustrated most clearly within the Adverse Childhood Experiences (ACEs) movement. This is a movement that recognises the long-lasting effect that trauma can have, and most significantly that which is experienced in childhood. This is a movement that is being championed right here in Scotland, UK. There have been numerous large conferences and seminars across the country working to shape a new paradigm in this field.

Furthermore, there are people building compassion into other key areas: organisations are working within the prison systems bringing trauma informed practice and understanding to make rehabilitation possible and reduce reoffending, whilst supporting families on the outside to mitigate the trauma of the children whose parents are in prison. I was present at an inspiring talk from an organisation which is implementing compassionate change to their housing system through building relationships with their tenants and subsequently preventing homelessness. In schools, trauma informed practice is becoming more commonplace including a paradigm shift beginning in the understanding of additional support needs of all kinds, meaning we are supporting the children and young people to access education in a way that demonstrates compassion and understanding for their needs, their home life, and circumstances, and recognising how that can impact their ability to access education.

It gives me great hope to see this happening in my own country where we are building compassion and love into our structures; it helps us to see the person in front of us as a suffering human the same as ourselves. What a powerful difference that makes as we view systems and people holistically and work together rather than pigeon holing and pathologizing the people we support and work with.

Love begins with us, and it starts with the simplest of gestures; a smile, a hug, picking up something someone else has dropped, a kind word. I tell my children I love them every day, I hug them, and show them what love is in many ways, and I know I'm not the only one. I can see the world is changing, and there is a new generation that truly is bringing in the culture of love that was started in the sixties, when people started waking up to a new ideal and the real possibility that we can build our world on love, not war.

Notes

Guided Message

If love is all you need then you are off to a good start as you are indeed filled with love and operate on that level. This world is changing, and fast, and you all need to speed up to keep up with it. This causes some stress for you but stay centred in love and all will be well. It is only a matter of time before everything changes for the better and that is what is happening now. The process has begun and we see this in the chaos that is visible in the world. It is all coming to the surface to be seen and cleared out, to make way for the new paradigm of love. This is all that we hope for as we watch over you, that you may be surrounded in love, in a world filled with it and so it shall be!

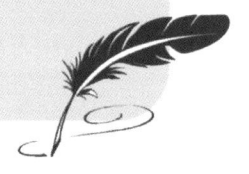

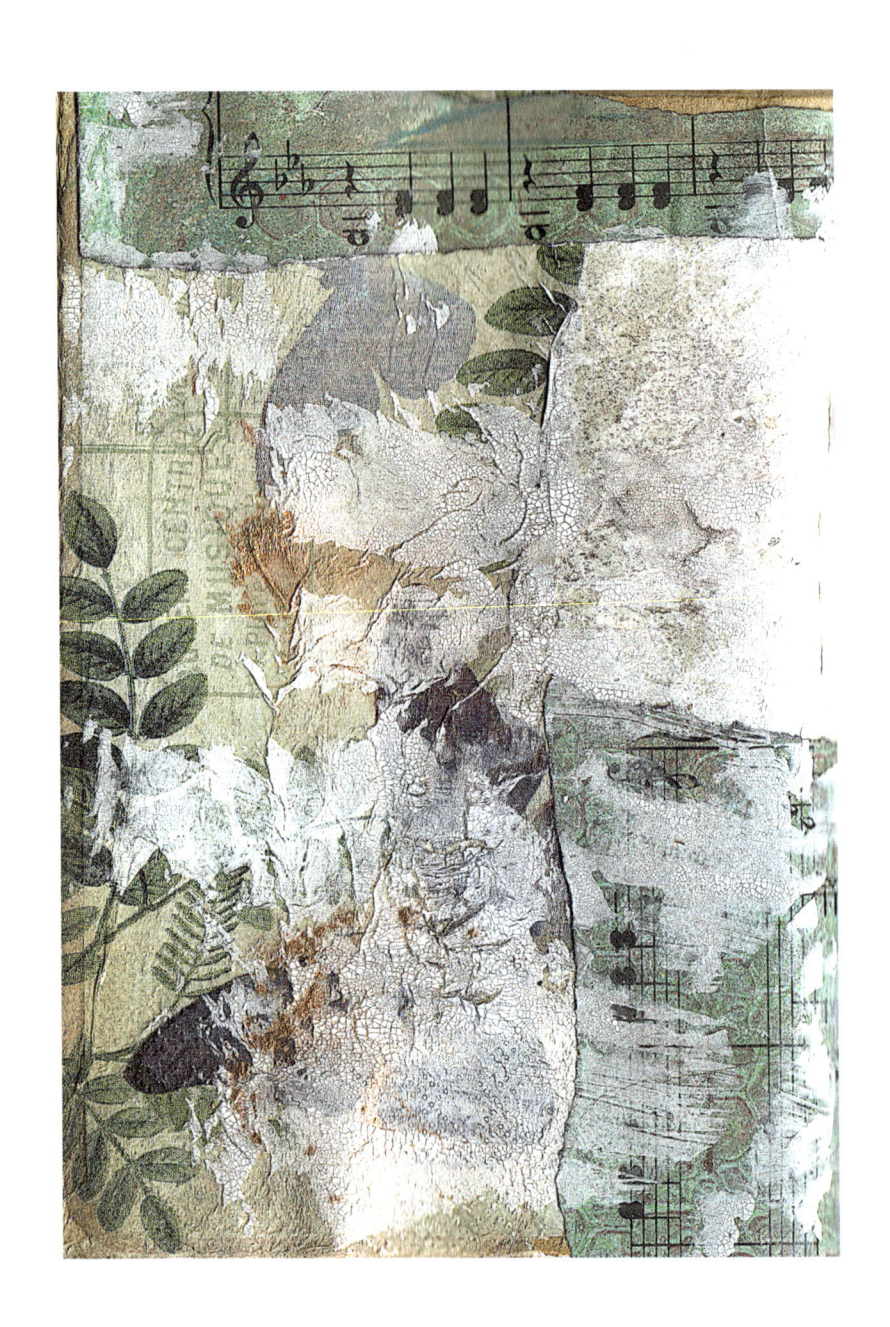

The Theory of Singing

As a traditional storyteller singing is a part of my practice as well as my passion, and my work. I love learning traditional ballads, children's lullabies and rhymes and other interesting contemporary pieces that come up along the way. I have a theory about singing and where the voice for singing comes from, and this includes the voice I use for telling stories.

Trauma affects us all differently, and what made it clear to me that my trauma was getting in the way of things was when I stopped being able to sing and when I stopped telling stories. I don't remember if it happened suddenly or if it was a gradual process. Trauma affects my ability to properly remember the timelines of when things occurred, so I can't be sure exactly how this went down.

As I recall, around the time it began to happen I was doing a lot of driving for my other work and had a long commute. I would listen to podcasts and music and of course, like anyone might, I would sing along to my favourite songs. Sometimes I would use the time to rehearse a story I was learning or practice singing a ballad. I'm really shy about anyone hearing me rehearse so the car is an ideal place.

Then one day it began. I opened my mouth to sing and nothing would come out. I felt my throat close and just shut down, and then I cried. I kept trying every day, but the same thing happened and most of the time it was the tears that would come. I spent many commutes weeping at my steering wheel and who knows what the other drivers must have thought if they turned and saw me. Somehow, I would pull myself together for work and get on with the day, but the cracks were showing, and it was only a matter of time before the dam would break.

What was happening here was that I had spent so many years coping with my trauma and feelings and putting on a brave face that now I was breaking. I felt deeply overwhelmed and was drowning in a depth of sorrow and despair that I never thought was possible. I was so far down in this pit of sadness I could see no light. I hurt on every level of my emotional being and I lived only to make it to the end of the day. There were a few different things that were happening in my life at that time that were contributing to my difficulties that I won't go into here. I guess they may be for my difficult second book! But what I did know was that my morning tears were not a normal response to all of that, and I needed help.

   My voice had shrivelled into a dry little walnut where death resided, that sat at the top of my oesophagus and blocked the passage of healing notes and words flowing to my body, towards my heart. My pain had grown so great that my connection with the creative part of me that bridges with the stories and the songs was gone. The element that makes them come alive, the desire, the spirit, the dance, the heart. There was no heart left in me, it was broken, I was lost and full of fear. I felt utterly adrift with no shred of hope. What I did have was some knowledge and the smallest piece of courage.

   I've worked in and around mental health for a long time, so I was certain where I needed to be. When I walked into the counselling centre to speak to someone, I knew this was my last chance. It was do or die and a desperate cry for help. Unsurprisingly, they put me on a waiting list, and to cut a long story short, after waiting for months I received a short course of counselling, after which they referred me on to another service for longer term in-depth therapy. Three years after that self-referral I told a story and sang a ballad at an event, and two years after that, therapy ended, and I had found not only my voice again but my Self.

THE THEORY OF SINGING

What I discovered on that journey I can only say is true for me, but I believe that the voice I use for telling stories and singing is the voice that comes not only from my heart but from my soul. When I'm participating in either of those activities, I am accessing the deepest aspect of me. I am consciously connecting inside of myself with the most creative and passionate part of who I am. I've felt it happen when I'm facilitating as well. Back then, I was so shrouded in despair that I had lost all access to that principal piece. I had shut down, and it was the most terrible time of my life, and yet somehow, I managed to not give up. As I've said before, my work keeps me going, and being connected with other people helps me as well. I hate to feel isolated and alone, so I also kept in good contact with some of my best supports; certain people in my life I found it easier to talk to. They were a lifeline for me and were generous with their patience and time in supporting me with a talking space.

Acceptance was also key in this this. I had to put one foot in front of the other and lean into the pain. What this means is that during therapy I allowed my despair to step over the threshold and through the door where I looked it square in the face. She was not a pretty sight. I learnt to understand her wretchedness because she was a big part of me, and as I did so, it initiated a softening and an opening up, and my voice tentatively began to come back. I would periodically test it out and sometimes it would crack, or I would just cry, until one day, I sang out, and then I cried again! It was an achingly long time before I could properly sing again but when I did, I found my voice had changed. It was deeper and more resonant. I could feel into my Self more, and as I told that first story, I understood my part within it in a different way.

We're all a part of the stories we tell whether we're telling a story about ourselves or not, because we're all connected, and when we sing, we are baring that truest part of ourselves, the most vulnerable and the most beautiful. Perhaps, this is why so many people shy away from singing because to do so will reveal so much of who they are, and not everyone is ready to do that or feels safe enough.

For me, singing feels like bringing my soul forward and connecting with my higher self, the element that is looking out for me. The part that steered me to counselling and gave me the courage to embrace my inner child, and her wretchedness. I think it's the closest thing I know to joy, and that might be the reason why sometimes when I sing, I cry.

Notes

Guided Message

O Dear One! When we hear you sing our own hearts fill with joy and great love for you! Singing is an expression that uses all elements of your body, and your soul so when they combine it is indeed a heavenly choir all of its own. Connecting to this part of you is incredibly healing as the sound you make that comes out with your body, heals the body within. This is why you all love to sing so much, why singing is such a huge part of all cultures. It is known and understood at an unconscious level that this is a vital part of your daily practice for health, healing, and wellbeing. Come back to it more and embrace your beautiful voice. Join with others and make your voices sing together in their harmonies and beguile each other with your music. We are listening intently and with great anticipation for the music you will bring.

MUSICIANS
OF BREMEN

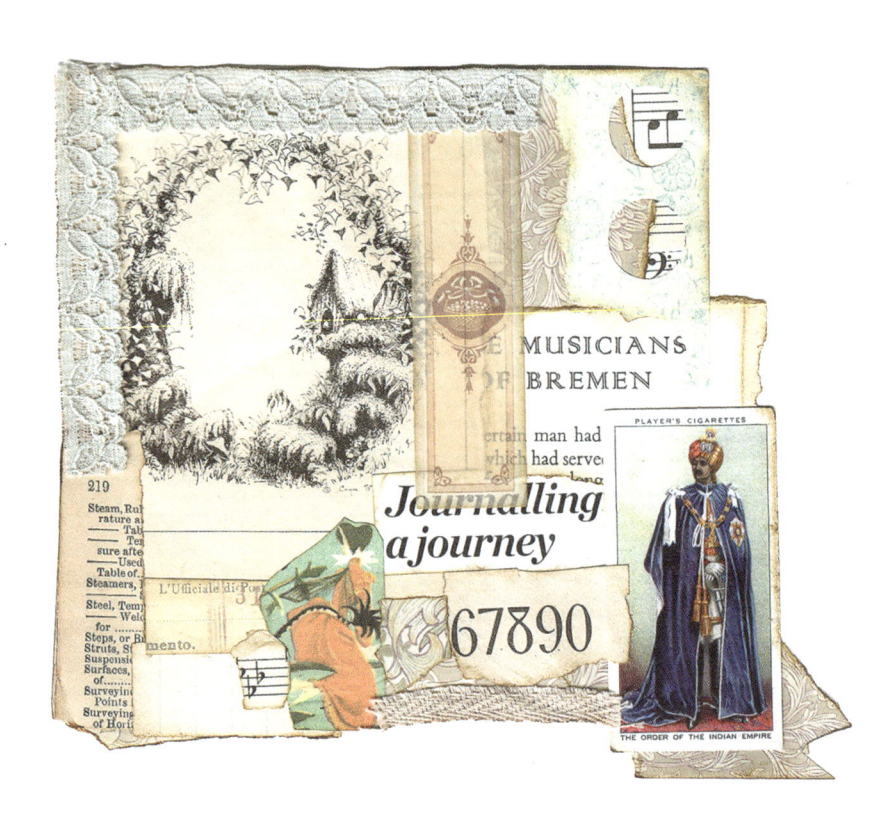

Journalling a journey

67890

THE ORDER OF THE INDIAN EMPIRE

Treatment and Recovery

It's been almost four weeks since they first put the Chemo into my arm through a PICC line, which is a permanent line inserted into my upper arm so they can administer repeated doses without wrecking the veins on the back of my hand with a canula every time. Showering is tricky as I can't get it wet, and we don't have a bath.

It's been almost four weeks of vomiting and nausea with one emergency hospital visit and a home visit from the GP who finally prescribed anti-sickness tablets that worked, although I was still sick a few times after that, and as recently as this morning.

It's been almost four weeks since I saw my Oncologist who I saw again yesterday, and she told me that they had in fact only given me a fifty percent dose of the Chemo, and showed no reaction when I told her of my horrific experience of the last few weeks as I sat in front of her barely able to lift my head as a sudden rush of sickness, exhaustion and flu type symptoms had come over me that morning but I didn't want to miss the appointment.

TREATMENT AND RECOVERY

It's been almost four weeks since I said yes to the Chemo treatment even though I've spent my whole adult life saying I would never have Chemo if I got cancer. However, something told me I should get it and so I followed my inner guidance on that, it's never steered me wrong. By the time I was four days into the treatment and sitting in the ambulance I insisted on the chemo being removed as soon as possible.

I felt like I had a parasite on my arm. You see they attach the Chemo bag to you so you can take it home and you don't have to stay in hospital. How convenient, although patients do fare better at home. I could not wait for it to be removed and by that point I was absolute in my feelings about Chemo and I knew I would not be continuing with the treatment. The following three weeks were nothing short of torture, and I hadn't even been given the full dose!

I'm glad I had the treatment though. Now I have more of an understanding of what cancer patients go through and just how debilitating and hard it is. I lost at least five kilograms in weight as much of the time I was either vomiting or feeling nauseous, so could barely eat. Being in hospital was mostly a horrible experience during that emergency visit and I may write about that another time.

JOURNALING A JOURNEY

I believe I had to go through that experience to understand the pain and suffering but I also believe I don't have to continue it. In the last twenty years I've tried to avoid putting chemicals into my body, apart from alcohol which I've been clear of for six years now, another story for another time. I've always leaned toward natural and organic methods in my cooking and lifestyle. So, flooding my body with what can only be described as a poison is counterintuitive to all my beliefs. It's not that I'm perfect by any means, I like my cake and junk food! But this just feels a step too far for me, and I can't bear the thought of putting rounds and rounds of that chemical into my body.

It's difficult to tell people this but I do now have a plan, and I am following a strict dietary protocol and have found other more natural ways to support my body and get rid of this tumour. I feel much more confident and positive about this, and I look forward to the Chemo symptoms going away, although the information they give you says that some symptoms can last for up to a year.

I must stress that this is a decision that's right for me and has always felt right but I still think Chemo can be right for others, and I personally know people who have had Chemo and it's cured their cancer. It's just

TREATMENT AND RECOVERY

not for me, and I have every respect for those who take it. I strongly feel we must do what feels right for ourselves. I know people may think I'm crazy, but I feel the opposite, and I think it's interesting to find that I'm following my initial belief that I would not have Chemo if I got cancer.

It's been almost four weeks since they put a needle in my arm and flooded my body with poison and I'm still vomiting. I won't be doing this again and I'm excited and interested to see what results I get from these other methods.

One of these other methods is based on the theory that your body needs the correct balance of minerals in order for it to function effectively. After being tested, I was shown the areas of imbalance in my body and was given a selection of minerals to address this. I'm updating this piece of writing as this book goes to publishing, and I'm delighted to report that having been tested again in the last week, my body's mineral balance has improved. I'll continue to take their supplements and hope this continues. I'm also drinking daily super nutrition smoothies which are tailored to my needs and am following a strict low carb, no sugar, high nutrition diet. I had my first CT scan three weeks ago which showed that the tumour is now stable and has not spread further. This is incredible news as prior to Christmas its growth was aggressive and progressively more painful week by week.

  Although I am still in a lot of pain, it's a different kind of pain and I feel like I'm in more of a holding pattern rather damage control. I've always felt connected with nature and more drawn to using natural methods and products. Therefore, I'll keep following these protocols and travelling in this direction as it feels more positive for me.

Notes

Guided Message

The suffering is a phase which no one wants to go through, and when it happens it causes such torment and upset for everyone. It has a purpose and serves to enhance and highlight one's inner strengths and show you what you never knew about yourself. This is hard to hear for most people as the suffering also feels so unfair. It is a horrific experience to go through and not one that we wish to see happen. You do have immense strength as do others who are going through similar experience, and we gather around you with as much support and healing as we can to ease your pain. As you begin to recover you can remember these incredible moments of strength where you have had to dig the deepest you have ever done and be proud of what you have achieved. This serves you well for your future, and do not underestimate what benefits may yet come from this down the line. It is impossible to know what may yet come but when one is put through these kinds of experience, we can assure you it is only for the greater good. You are a wonderful human being, and we commend you in the highest and gaze forward into your future with great hope and love.

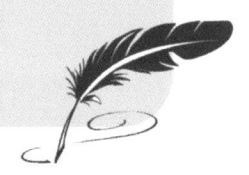

Design the life *you* want

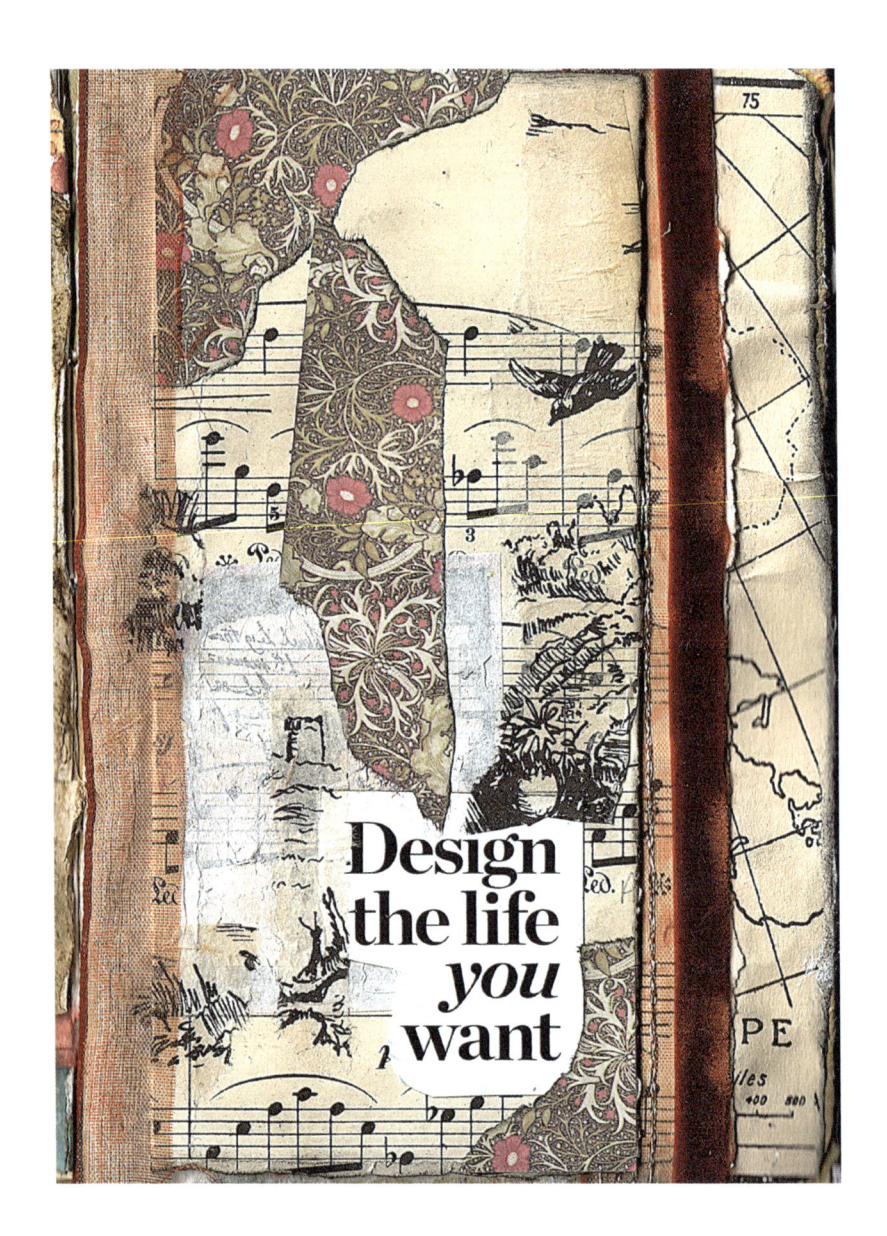

The Motivation

I have no idea if I'll be able to clear the cancer, but I know I must try, and since chemo neither agrees with my body or my ideals then I need to find other ways. I've done a ton of research as have friends of mine who feel a similar way. There is plenty of information out there about alternative ways to combat and prevent cancer, it's just that none of it is in the mainstream. We don't hear about other ways to cure cancer except for chemotherapy, and the reality is, the stats for survival and longevity vary broadly depending on who is reporting them, and are often low, much lower than I expected. As I've discovered, the side effects of chemo are brutal and can last for years, and it makes sense to me that there must be ways other than flooding our body with poison to prevent and cure cancer. Apparently, cancer cells are growing in our bodies all the time; it's just a case of whether they go rogue and start mutating, and there are reasons why they do, most often linked to diet and lifestyle.

THE MOTIVATION

I'm tired and I'm in pain a lot of the time so it's been helpful to have people around me who are suggesting and highlighting alternative pathways to healing. I've just received a batch of minerals from an organisation I had been to when I was pregnant with my first son seventeen years ago. Back then they cured me of a chronic skin condition that I'd been suffering from for many years that doctors and dermatologists couldn't figure out. So, when my cousin reminded me of them, I thought I would go back for some advice. I've just finished a three day fast and in the last six weeks have completed another three days, as well as a forty-five hour and a thirty-six hour fast. I also do intermittent fasting and follow a Ketogenic diet, which has no sugar and very low carbohydrates. Due to my research, I believe all of this is not only preventative for cancer but can also shrink tumours. I was surprised when I didn't find the three days fast difficult except for the desire to continue the routine of eating, I missed eating! It could be that I've got used to fasting and I also eat very little these days, plus my diet has become very refined.

I'm taking one intervention from the hospital which is Immunotherapy. It's a fairly new therapy that involves putting chemicals in the body that trigger and amplify the immune system to help it recognise and attack cancer cells, and so far, the side effects are minor. I've heard some positive reviews about it from nurses and patients I've met, so I'm hopeful it makes a difference.

I've been optimistic and positive about my diagnosis right from the start, and I don't know why. It feels like I have an automatic driving force inside that is moving me forward without my even trying. I have a strong spiritual practice so I guess I would say that it's my soul that I'm connecting with, and it's providing me with a reassurance that's giving me the strength to keep going.

When the consultant told me how ill I was, there were two distinct emotions that gripped me at the same time: I started to sob at the harsh reality, whilst simultaneously experiencing a surge of adrenaline and a sort of a thrill as I faced my mortality. It's not every day you're told you have a limited span of life left and to start counting. To be clear, that was not how she put it to me. For a while I felt like I was standing outside of myself observing this amazing thing we call life, and death, and it was kind of cool. But we're all going to die at some point, aren't we? It's just that bit more definitive when the doc tells you that Death is already travelling your way and sharpening his scythe.

THE MOTIVATION

I've always been an adrenaline seeker, so I suppose that moment was just another form of excitement, like climbing the top of a mountain or riding bikes super-fast down steep mountains, climbing ice walls or jumping out of a plane at ten thousand feet, all of which I've done. My bucket list looks very different from a lot of others I know as I've already done a great deal of things in my life. I'm not interested in bucket lists, the last twenty-three years of my life I've been doing whatever I want anyway. My desire now is to travel more but other than that I'm perfectly happy with what I've got, and I couldn't ask for more. After living the largest portion of my life with the symptoms of trauma there is nothing I like better than the feeling of peace in my mind, and I thank God that I completed the therapy for that before this happened to enable me to be calm enough to handle things as well as I am.

I'll keep writing, and praying, and meditating and putting one foot in front of the other. It's a slow process but then, isn't everything good in life worth waiting for?

Disclaimer: I am not an expert in any of this and all views are my own. The diets I describe work for me, and I don't recommend fasting without checking with your

GP first. *The link below is to support the reader in further research if they desire.*

What Is Autophagy? 8 Amazing Benefits Of Fasting That Will Save Your Life

Dr Sten Ekberg

https://www.youtube.com/watch?v=XCvUf9WU4qI

Notes

Guided Message

The wisdom you seek is always within but if you are looking for validation upon any subject then look for the signs. All around you the universe is speaking to show you in different ways whether you are facing the right direction. We do not weep with you when you die to this earthly plane but rather, we rejoice as you are coming home. There is nothing to fear in death except that we understand the sadness and the loss of the lives you have led here on this plane, they are hard to let go. You want to prolong your time here and enjoy more of the life you have made and that is ok and makes sense. We support you in that and hope you can find the ways to do this. We know how attached you become to these lives but are here to remind you that there is so much more to this universe than you can see. It is all around you, these magic and different dimensional planes. Dip in and out of it with your intuition to seek guidance in matters of importance and take heart knowing that we will never steer you wrong. We love you with all the power of the universe and send you the healing you need to continue your path.

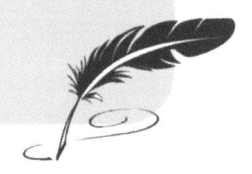

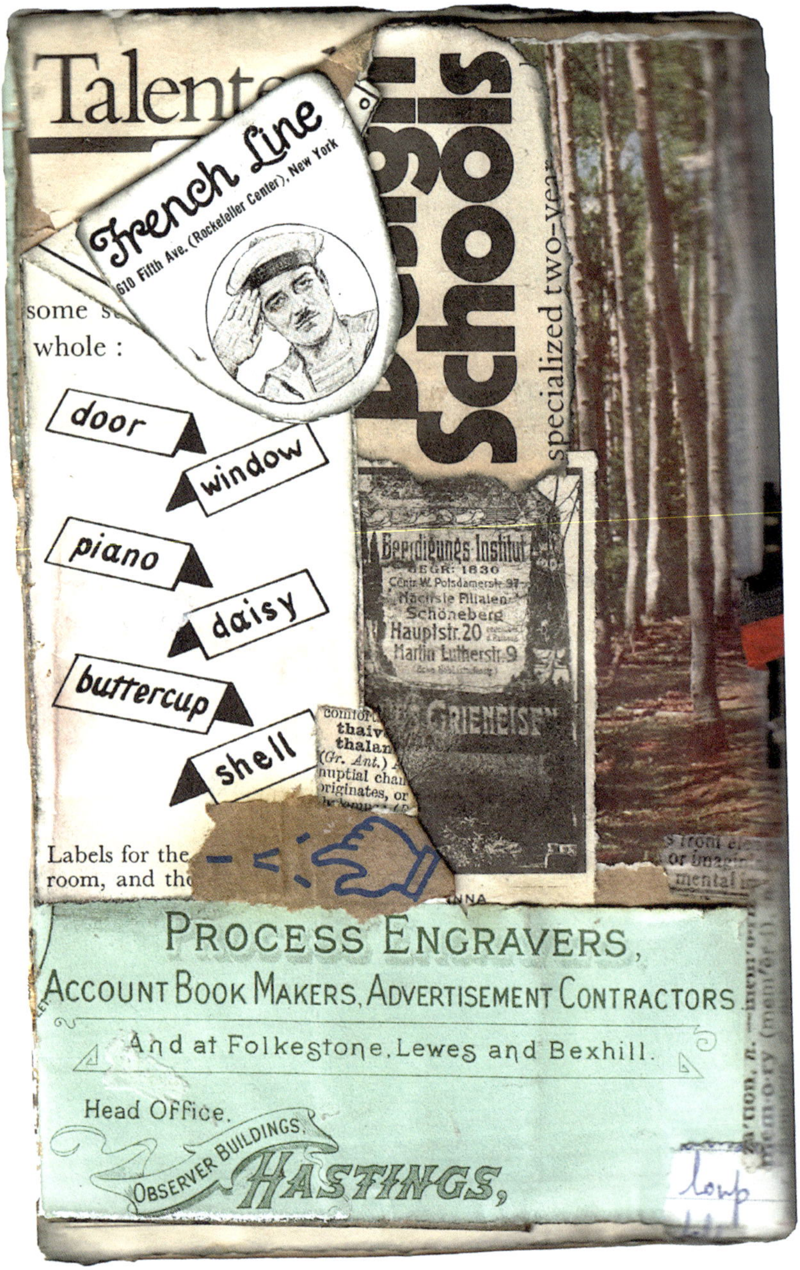
Talent
French Line
610 Fifth Ave. (Rockefeller Center), New York
Schools
specialized two-year
some
whole :
door
window
piano
daisy
buttercup
shell
Schöneberg
Hauptstr. 20
Martin Lutherstr. 9
thaiv
thalan
(Gr. Ant.)
nuptial cha
originates, or
Labels for the
room, and the
PROCESS ENGRAVERS,
ACCOUNT BOOK MAKERS, ADVERTISEMENT CONTRACTORS.
And at Folkestone, Lewes and Bexhill.
Head Office.
OBSERVER BUILDINGS,
HASTINGS,

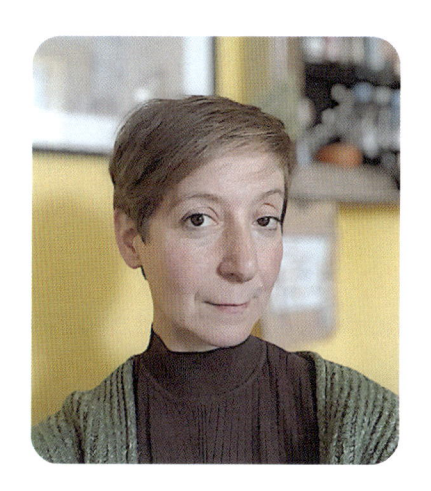

About The Author

~ Wendy Woolfson ~

Wendy Woolfson is a professional storyteller and facilitator, specialising in supporting families and professionals to work collaboratively in meeting the needs of vulnerable children and young people through storytelling and trauma sensitive practice. She is the creator of the Out of Harm Toolkit which supports understanding of self-harm. She works in small therapeutic groups for people to explore stories, including their own. Wendy has more than 17 years of storytelling experience, is a Solution Focused Brief Therapy Practitioner and holds a Professional Diploma in Therapeutic Life Story Work. She currently works in social care for a Scottish charity.

She is a mixed media artist who creates and binds artisanal books and ephemera in the style of vintage junk journals. Wendy works primarily with paper and mixed media to produce junk journals, ephemera and other stationery and paper fold type items. She uses inks, paints and largely vintage materials and found objects. She especially loves using vintage papers to produce work that is nostalgic, reminiscent and thought provoking. Stories enter into her work in a variety of ways and often provide a thread of story and mood throughout the pieces. Wendy frequently finds a phrase or word that prompts her; something that touches an emotional point within her and she works intuitively from there. In this way her work is largely autobiographical.

JOURNALING A JOURNEY

If you want to find out more about Wendy and her work, you can contact her through her website, or follow her on social media - see her Linktree or scan the QR code below:

https://linktr.ee/wendywoolfson

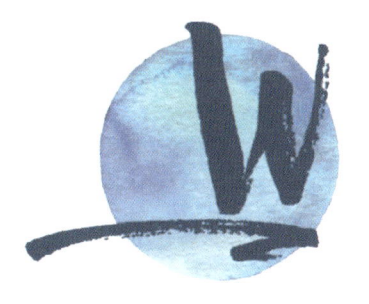

Acknowledgements

Murray for your unending love, caring and kindness, my heart and soul connection, for tending to my every need, I love you without end. My darling children, Harry and Angus for their patience, courage, and wicked humour!

Gaz, or rather Dr Gary, you have given so much and made such a difference, where would we be without you?

Fiona and Graeme for your love, support, and time you've taken to help us.

My brothers, Peter, Mark, and Giles, I love you so much, thank you for being here for me in all your different ways.

Jessica, my darling cousin, my sister, thank you for your love and your amazing support.

My dear friend Jenny, your love and support, your friendship without question and your delicious food!

Russell and Roisin thank you for your love and support, great food and finding freezers!

Alison and Tiffany, your spiritual guidance and love has been a strong and necessary foundation for me to stay grounded and optimistic.

Denise and Roger for your guidance and supplements and your friendship and love.

Sally, Jeanette, Georgia, Tania, Kate, Lizanne, Karen, Isobel, Susan, Colvil, thank you for your friendship, love, and support.

The Book Whisperers, my friends, for your incredible support and guidance creating and publishing this book.

Everyone on my social media who have constantly sent me so many messages of love and support that have really buoyed me up in hard times.

I give the last word to my therapist Kirstin, without whose gentle guidance I don't believe I'd be here today. Little Wendy is very grateful to you.

Thanks to all the amazing people who so kindly supported me on Kickstarter, you made a real difference!

Alan Fitchet	Deborah Hofman
Alastair McIver	Denise Wickings
Allison Galbraith	Donna Campbell
Andrew Remes	Ethne Woldman
Ann Stoddart	Fiona Lees
Anne Ellis	Fiona Wright
Arturo Cruz	Georgia Wolfson
Belinda Cohen	Giles Woolfson
Brittany Tilley	Graham Darnell
Carl Pickard	Guy Clayton
Catrin Evans	Ian Hopley
Claire Coia	Iona Kewney
Claire Obermark	Jane Mather
Colin Wood	Jean McClure
Dahlia Remes	Jean Edmiston
Daisy Richardson	Jeremy Martin
Daniel Berman	Jessica Gladys Wolfson
David Moran	Joe Graham

John Kenda
Joy Bain
Juan Mejia
Karen Oliver
Kate frame
Kate Walker
Kavitha Ratnam
Lea Taylor
Leigh Oliver
Lena Sjöberg
Lesley O'Brien
Linda McCurrach
Lizanne Conway
Louise Welsh
Mandy O'Connor
Mark Gallagher
Mark Woolfson
Mary Turner Thomson
Michael Remes
Michael Williams

Morag Langley
Natalie Silverdale
Noona Owens
Pauline McLachlan
Pete Tobias
Peter Woolfson
Priya logan
Rachel Robbins
Renee Rosenmann
Rowan Morrison
Sally Seddon
Sandra Walls
Sarah MoonFlower
Sarah Cameron
Sheryl Randhawa
Shola Sharbakova Miller
Tamar Dresner
Tania Berlow
Tiffany Stephens
Tim Norman

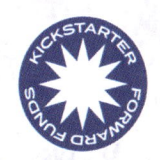

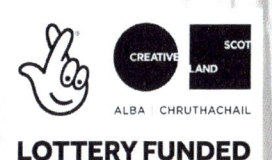

LOTTERY FUNDED

Know more than I tell...

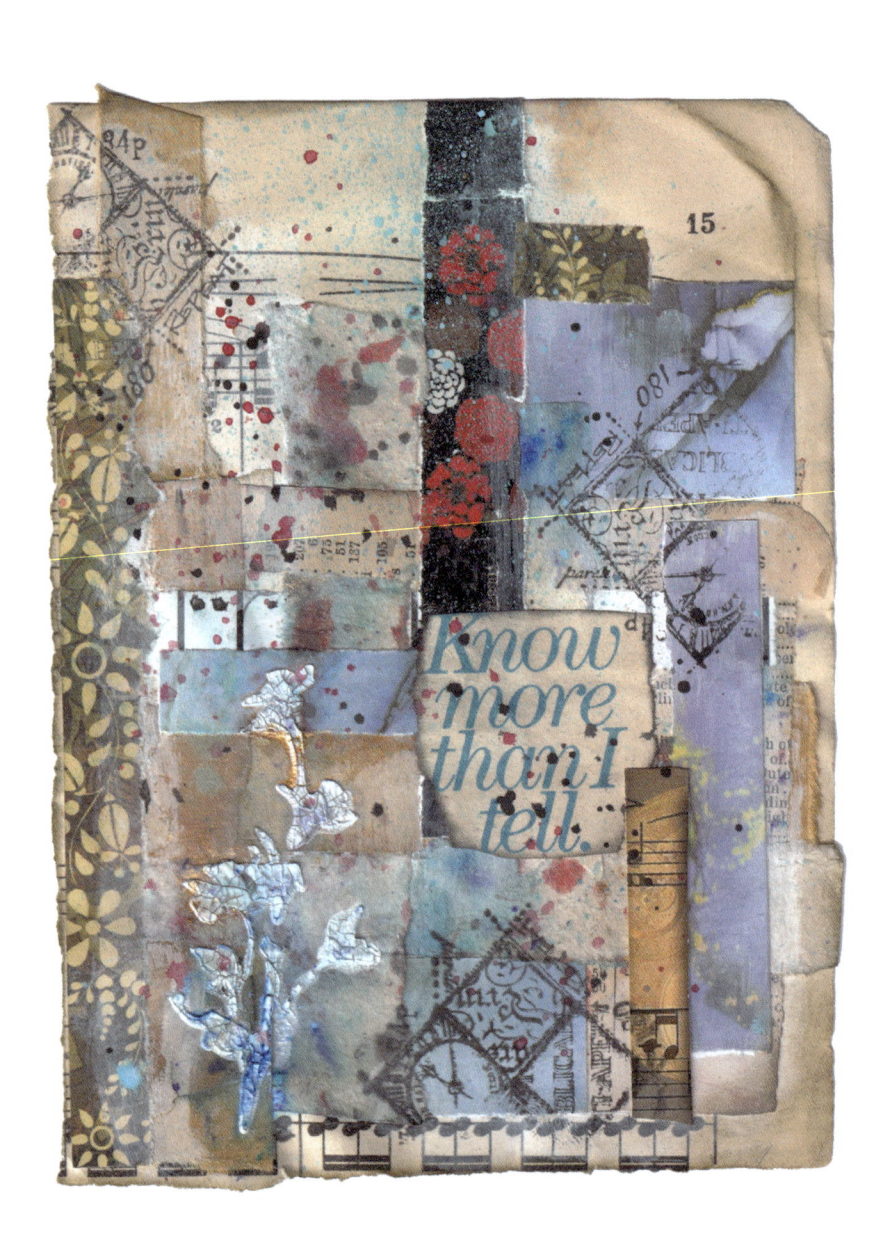

Journaling Pages

Journaling remains the mainstay of my wellbeing and mental health support, and I'd like to invite you to put pen to paper and write a few words in this book. It's okay to type on your computer if you prefer, maybe writing physically is difficult for you, that's okay. However you do it, the biology of transferring the written word through your hand can be cathartic and powerful, so I recommend doing it in any way you can.

I've provided some prompts here, and you can write something, draw, or doodle a picture, scratch marks, or shapes on the paper, whatever feels good. There are no rules, just enjoy transferring thought and image to paper and see what comes through. Allow the gentle and loving thoughts, the fearful and the dark, they all matter. If you make it a daily practice it becomes easier.

Notes

Prompt:
What am I grateful for today?

Notes

Prompt:
What does my soul need me to do today?

Notes

Prompt:
What kind things can I tell myself, or do for myself today?

Notes

Support and Helplines

Please don't struggle with your mental health on your own. Reach out to a friend or family member if you can, or sometimes talking to a stranger is easier. These are a few UK Based numbers you can call for good, confidential support.

Breathing Space

www.breathingspace.scot/

0800 83 85 87

Our advisors provide listening, information, and advice for people in Scotland feeling low, stressed or anxious.

Samaritans

www.samaritans.org/how-we-can-help/contact-samaritan/

Call 116 123

Whatever you're going through,
a Samaritan will face it with you.

We're here 24 hours a day, 365 days a year.

Childline

www.childline.org.uk/

0800 1111

Information, advice and support for
children and young people up to age 19.

Useful for parents to have a look at as well.

Parentline

www.children1st.org.uk/help-for-families/parentline-scotland/

Do you feel like you're at the end of your tether?

Children 1st Parentline is here for you and your family.

If you live in Scotland call 08000 28 22 33 free, Browse our website for advice and support, or start a webchat.

Young Minds

www.youngminds.org.uk

Whether you want to understand more about how you're feeling and find ways to feel better, or you want to support someone who's struggling, we can help.

For young people, parents, and workers

Papyrus

www.papyrus-uk.org

Are you, or is a young person you know, not coping with life? For confidential suicide prevention advice contact HOPELINE247

Phone - 0800 068 4141

Text - 07860 039967

Email - pat@papyrus-uk.org

Self-Harm Support

www.wendywoolfson.co.uk/out-of-harm

FREE downloadable Toolkit for professionals and public to gain understanding of self-harm plus a Conversation Guide to develop a language for talking to young people about self-harm, to build confidence and lessen fear.

References

Maslow's Hierarchy of Needs

https://en.wikipedia.org/wiki/Maslow's_hierarchy_of_needs

An idea in psychology proposed by American psychologist Abraham Maslow in his 1943 paper "A Theory of Human Motivation" in the journal Psychological Review.[1] Maslow subsequently extended the idea to include his observations of humans' innate curiosity. His theories parallel many other theories of human developmental psychology, some of which focus on describing the stages of growth in humans.

Daughter Detox, Peg Streep

https://pegstreep.com/about-daughter-detox-recovering-from-an-unloving-mother-and-reclaiming-your-life/#!

A self-help book based in science, the result of more than a decade of research, Daughter Detox offers the daughters of unloving mothers vital information, guidance, and real strategies for healing from childhood experiences, and building genuine self-esteem.

The Promise

https://thepromise.scot/

The Promise is that Scotland's children and young people will grow up loved, safe and respected.

Adverse Childhood Experiences (ACEs) Scotland

https://www.gov.scot/publications/adverse-childhood-experiences-aces

Our work to prevent and reduce the negative impact of childhood adversity and trauma.

What Is Autophagy?

8 Amazing Benefits Of Fasting That Will Save Your Life

Dr Sten Ekberg

https://www.youtube.com/watch?v=XCvUf9WU4qI

Notes

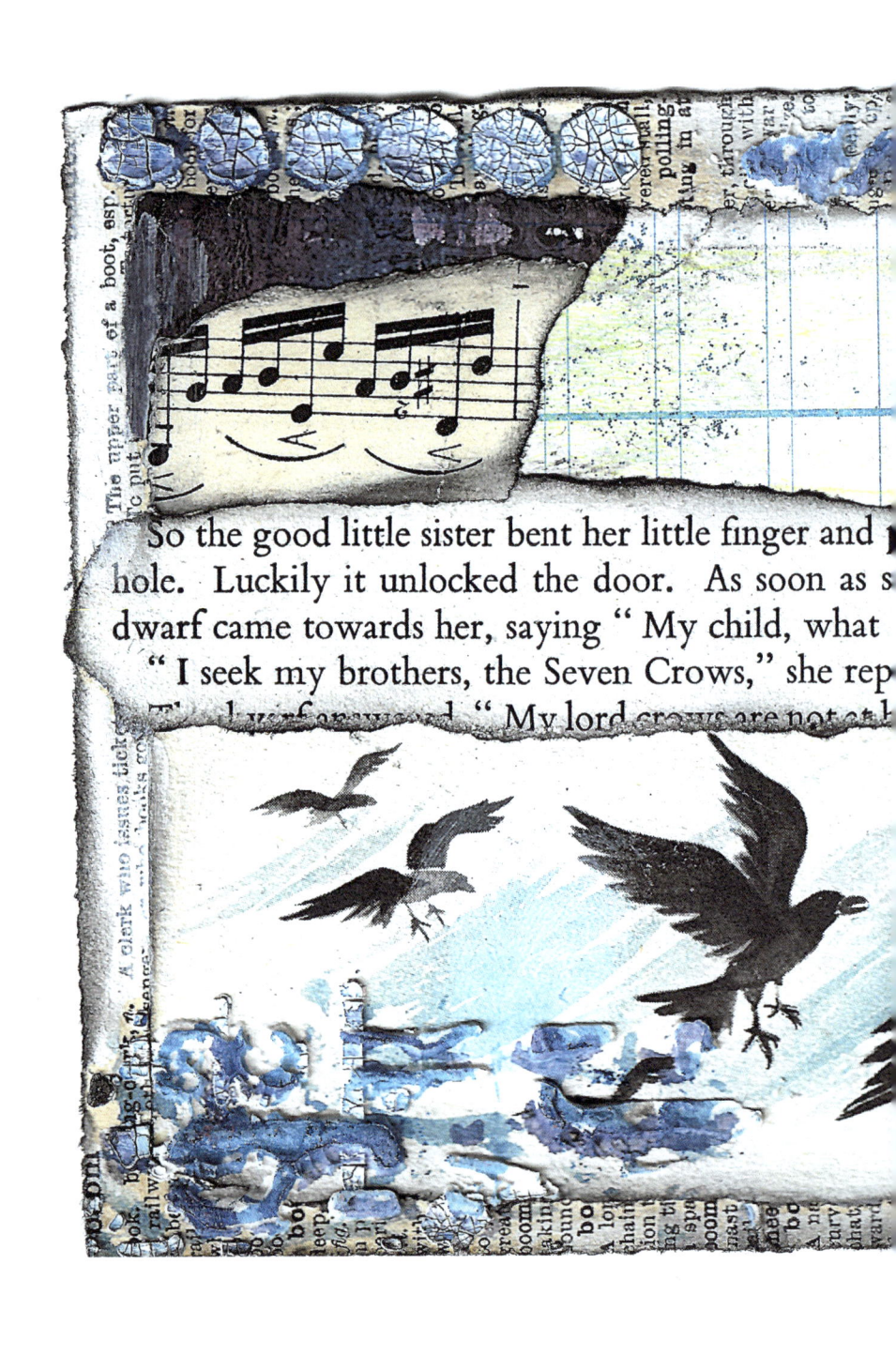

So the good little sister bent her little finger and
hole. Luckily it unlocked the door. As soon as s
dwarf came towards her, saying " My child, what
" I seek my brothers, the Seven Crows," she rep

to the key-
red, a little
seek?"

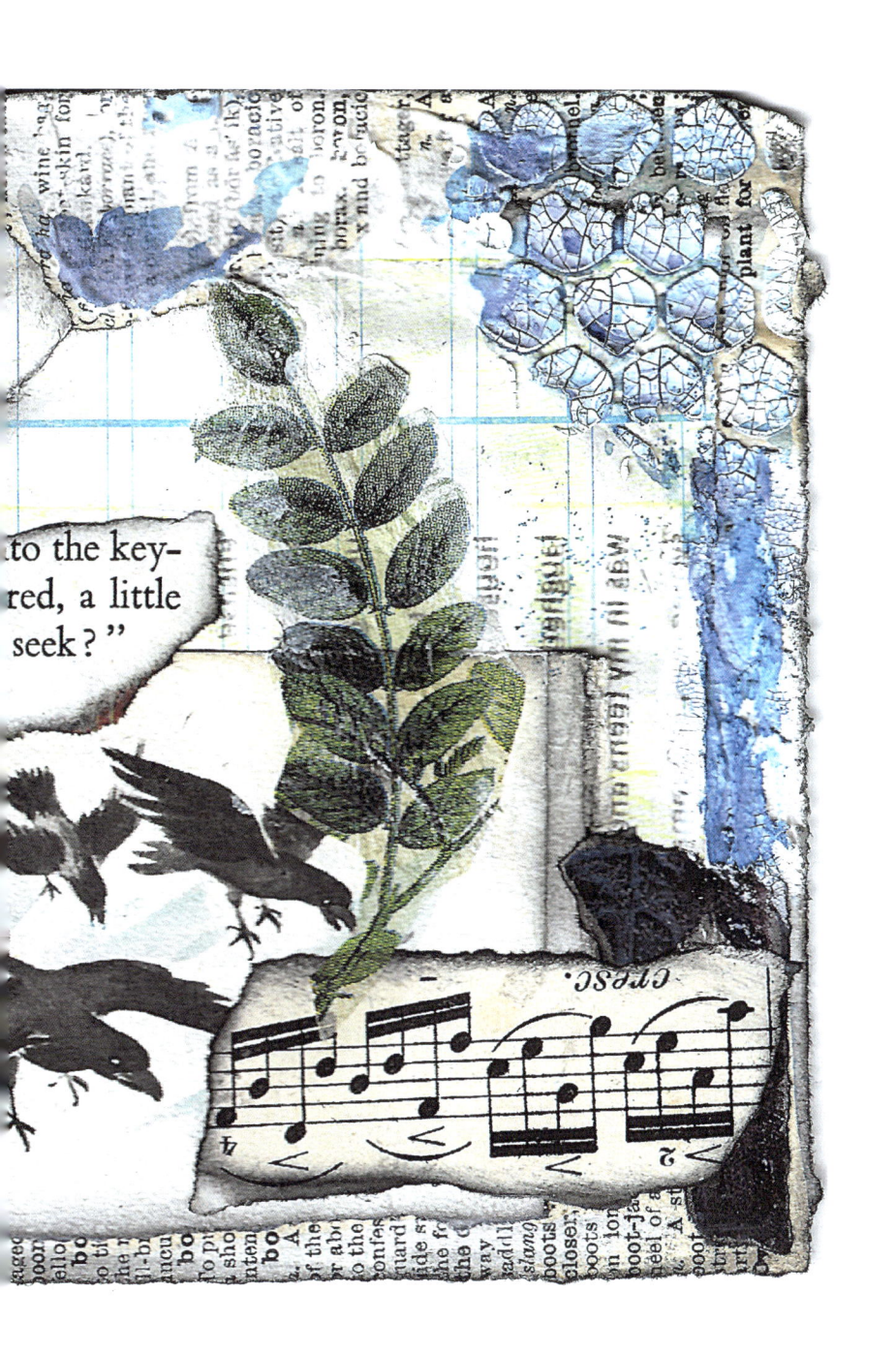

Transformation

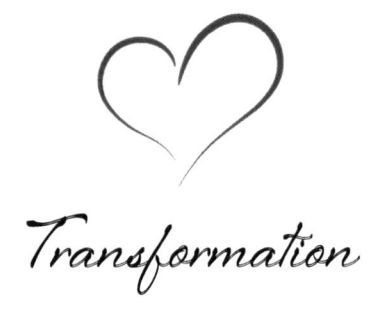

Pain moves through you
as light casts brilliance
on a dark space
and illuminates
what can't be seen.

Illuminates dark corners
for others to see.
Reveals your true nature.

When the suffering is over
You will feel grateful
As you step into your soul, fully.

Your energy encourages others
As you too have been encouraged

For this is how it works.
Rejoice in your resilience and strength.

Printed in Great Britain
by Amazon

5dd6e41e-f46a-41f5-b268-cc30e7f9bc27R01